ADULT HIV/AIDS TREATMENT POCKET GUIDE 2016

John G. Bartlett, MD
Professor Emeritus
Johns Hopkins University School of Medicine

Joel E. Gallant, MD, MPH
Medical Director of Specialty Services
Southwest CARE Center
Adjunct Professor of Medicine
Johns Hopkins University School of Medicine

Paul A. Pham, Pharm.D. BCPS
Managing Partner
Westview Urgent Care MediCenter
Clinical Associate Professor
University of Maryland School of Pharmacy

Important Information for the Users of This Pocket Guide

This document is provided as an information resource for physicians and other health care professionals to assist in the appropriate treatment of patients with HIV/AIDS. Recommendations for care and treatment change rapidly, and opinion can be controversial; therefore, physicians and other health care professionals are encouraged to consult other sources, especially FDA approved manufacturers' package inserts, and confirm the information contained on these tables. The individual health care professional should use his/her best medical judgment in determining appropriate patient care or treatment because no reference or guideline can trump provider judgment, based on individual patient issues, available resources, and updated information.

This pocket guide includes tables reflecting the authors' efforts to accurately report contemporary recommendation based largely on federal guidelines for HIV care and new developments by attendance at major scientific conferences and by systematic review of 42 relevant journals. Recommendations presented here are based largely on US federal guidelines for antiretroviral therapy for adults, pregnancy, prophylaxis and treatment of opportunistic infections, management of occupational exposure, management of co-infection with tuberculosis, hepatitis B, and hepatitis C, prevention of transmission, and management of sexually transmitted infections. Based on recent advances there has been substantial change in nearly all categories of care.

Inquiries, comments, and corrections about the Pocket Guide may be addressed to jgbartletthivguide@gmail.com

References for the Pocket Guide to HIV/AIDS Treatment

Primary Care: Primary Care Guidelines for the Management of Persons Infected with Human Immunodeficiency Virus: 2014 Update by the HIV Medicine Association of the Infectious Diseases Society of America. Aberg JA, et al. *Clin Infect Dis* 2014; 58:1-10.

Antiretroviral Agents for Adults (DHHS): 2015 Guidelines for the Use of Antiretroviral Agents in HIV-1-Infected Adults and Adolescents, May 19, 2015. Available at http://www.aidsinfo.nih.gov/guidelines/ and IAS-USA 2014 guidelines. *JAMA* 2014;312: 410

WHO Guidelines: See consolidated Strategic Information 2014 Guidelines for HIV Prevention, Diagnosis, Treatment and Care, July 2014 (http://www.who.int/hiv/pub/guidelines/keypopulations/en/)

Lipid Guidelines: 2013 ACC/AHA guideline on the assessment of cardiovascular risk: A report of the American College of Cardiology/American Heart Association Task Force on Practice Guideline. Stone NJ et al. Circulation 2014; 129 Suppl 2: S1-45

Antiretroviral Agents in Pregnancy 2015 DHHS: Recommendations for Use of Antiretroviral Drugs in Pregnant HIV-1-Infected Women for Maternal Health and Interventions to Reduce Perinatal HIV Transmission in the United States. August 6 2015. https://aidsinfo.nih.gov/guidelines/html/3/perinatal-guidelines/0#

Prevention and treatment of Opportunistic Infections: DHHS Guidelines for the Prevention and Treatment of Opportunistic Infections in HIV-Infected Adults and Adolescents. April 16, 2015. Available at http://aidsinfo.nih.gov/contentfiles/lvguidelines/Adult_OI.pdf

TB Prevention and Treatment: TB Guidelines for HIV/TB co-infection: CDC guidelines 2013 www.cdc.gov/tb/publications/guidelines/Treatment.htm. American Thoracic Society / CDC/IDSA Treatment of Tuberculosis. *MMWR* 2005;54 (RR-12):1-81;(RR-15):1-47; and (RR-17):1-14:4-44); *MMWR* 2009;58(RR-4:1-207) and (RR-5:1-207); *MMWR* 2010;59 (RR-5):1-25. Available at http://www.cdc.gov/tb/. see DHHS Opportunistic Infection Guidelines-April 16, 2015 edition section F

STD Prevention and Treatment: Sexually Transmitted Disease Treatment CDC 2015 Guidelines. CDC *MMWR Recomm and Rep* 2015; 64: 1-137. Available at http://www.cdc.gov/std/tg2015/tg-2015-print.pdf

HIV Prophylaxis with Occupational HIV Exposure: Updated U.S. Public Health Service Guidelines for the Management of Occupational Exposures to HIV and Recommendations for Postexposure Prophylaxis - see: PEP Quick Guide for Occupational Exposures, CDC, updated 2/2/14 http://nccc.ucsf.edu/clinical-resources/pep-resources/pep-quick-guide/; Kuhar DT Infect Control Epidemiol 2013; 34: 875-92

HIV management with Encyclopedic Coverage: New York State AIDS Institute Guidelines. http://guideline.gov/content.aspx?id=24037

Pre-Exposure Prophylaxis (PrEP): CDC guidelines for the prevention of HIV infection in-2014. http://www.cdc.gov/hiv/pdf/prepguidelines2014.pdf

Antiretroviral Drug Resistance Mutation and Testing: 2015 Stanford database and 2014 Recommendations of IAS-USA. *Top HIV Med* June/July. 2014;22:642 and http://hivdb.stanford.edu.

Vaccines for HIV-infected persons: 2015 CDC Recommendations. Kim DK Ann Intern Med 2015; 162: 214-223

HIV testing: 2015 CDC recommendations: Branson B. Curr HIV/AIDS Rep 2015;12:117-126

TABLE 1: **Drug and Treatment Information Resources**

Resource	Information and Source
AIDSInfo www.aidsinfo.nih.gov	DHHS Guidelines for ART in adults, pediatrics, and pregnancy
AETC www.aids-ed.org/aidsetc?page=cm-0D-0D	Clinical Manual for Management of the HIV-Infected Adult
AETC www.aids-ed.org	Training resources, slide sets, self study, and more
HIV InSite www.hivinsite.org	Knowledge base, drug interactions, global country profiles, and more
Johns Hopkins HIV Guide www.hopkins-hivguide.org	Clinical database, handheld HIV, publications, Q&A forum
Medscape HIV/AIDS www.medscape.com/hiv	News, conference coverage, drug interactions, reviews, Q&A, CME and more
National HIV/AIDS Clinicians Consultation Center www.nccc.ucsf.edu	AETC clinical resource, contact to warm line and PEPline
International AIDS Society-USA www.iasusa.org	CME, resistance mutation chart, cases
VA National HIV/AIDS Program www.hiv.va.gov	Information for providers and patients
International Training and Education Center on HIV www.go2itech.org	International AETC with training material
HIV Web Study depts.washington.edu/hivaids	University of Washington cases, tables, images
Stanford University HIV Drug Resistance Database hivdb.stanford.edu	Resistance mutations and interpretations
Clinical Care Options www.clinicaloptions.com/HIV.aspx	Reviews, CME, and conference summaries
New York State Department of Health AIDS Institute www.nyhealth.gov/diseases/aids/standards	Guidelines for treatment of HIV, opportunistic infections, laboratory monitoring, systemic reviews, PEP, PrEP
Integrated services for HIV, STDs, hepatitis and TB for IDU pts (MMWR 2015; 65 (rr 13): 1-37)	HIV, STD, HBV, HCV, TB services
HIV Testing [Panner N, CDC: CID 2014; 59: 875-82; MMWR 2014; 63: 537] www.cdc.gov/mmwr/pdf/rr/rr5514.pdf	CDC recommendations for HIV screening 2014
Clinical Care Options http://www.clinicaloptions.com/HIV.aspx	News, conference coverage, drug interactions, reviews, Q&A, CME
Up To Date www.uptodate.com	Comprehensive medical database Updated ID and AIDS info

TABLE OF CONTENTS

TABLE 2: **Abbreviations for Antiretroviral Agents and Classes**

Antiretroviral Agents and Classes	
ABC: Abacavir (*Ziagen*)	InSTI: Integrase strand transfer inhibitor
ATV: Atazanavir (*Reyataz*)	LPV/r: Lopinavir/ritonavir (*Kaletra*)
AZT or ZDV: Zidovudine (*Retrovir*)	MVC: Maraviroc (*Selzentry*)
"/c": Boosted with cobicistat (*Tybost*)	NFV: Nelfinavir (*Viracept*)
COBI: Cobicistat (*Tybost*)	NNRTI: Non-nucleoside reverse transcriptase inhibitor
ddI: Didanosine (*Videx*)	NRTI: Nucleoside reverse transcriptase inhibitor
d4T: Stavudine (*Zerit*)	NVP: Nevirapine (*Viramune*)
DLV: Delavirdine (*Rescriptor*)	PI: Protease inhibitor
DTG: Dolutegravir (*Tivicay*)	PI/r: PI boosted with RTV
DRV: Darunavir (*Prezista*)	/r: Boosted with Ritonavir (RTV) $\leq$ 400 mg/d
EFV: Efavirenz (*Sustiva*)	RAL: Raltegravir (*Isentress*)
EVG: Elvitegravir (*Vitekta*)	RPV: Rilpivirine (*Edurant*)
EI: Entry Inhibitor	RTV: Ritonavir (*Norvir*)
ENF: Enfuvirtide (*Fuzeon*, *T-20*)	SQV: Saquinavir (*Invirase*)
ETR: Etravirine (*Intelence*)	3TC: Lamivudine (*Epivir*)
FPV: Fosamprenavir (*Lexiva*)	TAF: Tenofovir alafenamide
FTC: Emtricitabine (*Emtriva*)	TDF: Tenofovir Disoproxil fumarate (*Viread*)
	TPV: Tipranavir (*Aptivus*)

TABLE 2: **Abbreviations Used in This Pocket Guide** *(cont.)*

Miscellaneous (cont.)	
ACTG: AIDS Clinical Trial Group	ESRD: End-stage Renal Disease
ADR: Adverse Drug Reaction	ETOH: Alcohol
ART: Antiretroviral Therapy	FBS: Fasting Blood Glucose
AUC: Area Under the Concentration-Time Curve	FDA: US Food and Drug Administration
bid: twice per day	G6PD: Glucose 6-Phosphate Dehydrogenase
biw: twice per week	HAV: Hepatitis A Virus
BMD: Bone Mineral Density	HBsAb: Hepatitis B surface Antibody
CBC: Complete Blood Count	HBsAg: Hepatitis B surface Antigen
CDC: Centers for Disease Control	HBV: Hepatitis B Virus
CK: Creatine Kinase Assay	HCV: Hepatitis C Virus
CMV: Cytomegalovirus	HAART: Highly Active Antiretroviral Therapy
CPE: CNS penetration score	HIVAN: HIV-Associated Nephropathy
CPS: Child-Pugh Score	HIV-2: a retrovirus related to HIV
CrCl: Creatinine Kinase Clearance	HPV: Human Papilloma Virus
D/M tropic virus: Virus that is either dual-tropic (able to enter the CD4 cell using either the CCR5 or CXCR4 coreceptor) or a mixed population of R5- and X4-tropic virus	HSV-1: Herpes Simplex Virus Type 1
DEXA: Dual Energy X-ray	HSV-2: Herpes Simplex Virus Type 2
DHHS: US Department of Health and Human Services	hs: bedtime (hour of sleep)
DOT: Directly Observed Therapy	IDSA: Infectious Disease Society of America
DRESS: Drug Rash with Eosinophilia and Systemic Symptoms	IGRA: Interferon Gamma Releasing Assay
Dx: Diagnosis	IM: Intramuscular
EC: Enteric Coated	IRIS: Immune Reconstitution Inflammatory syndrome
EE: Ethinyl Estradiol	IV: Intravenous
EIA: Enzyme Immunoassay	IVIG: Intravenous Immune Globulin

TABLE 2: **Abbreviations Used in This Pocket Guide** *(cont.)*

Miscellaneous (cont.)	
KS: Kaposi sarcoma	qid: four times per day
MAC: Mycobacterium avium complex	qm: monthly
MDRTB: Multidrug Resistant TB	qod: every other day
mo: month	qw: every week
MSM: Men who have sex with men	RAM: Resistance Associated Mutations
MTCT: Maternal to Child Transmission	R5 Tropic Virus: HIV strain that enters the CD4 cell using the CCR5 coreceptor
NAAT: Nucleic Acid Amplification Test	Rx: Treatment
nPEP: Non-Occupational Exposure Prophylaxis	SJS: Stevens-Johnson Syndrome
OI: Opportunistic Infection	soln: solution
PCP: *Pneumocystis* Pneumonia	std or SD: Standard (dose)
PCR: Polymerase Chain Reaction	STD: Sexually Transmitted Disease
PEP: Post-Exposure Prophylaxis	Sx: Symptoms
PGL: Peripheral Generalized Lymphadenopathy	TAM: Thymidine Analog Mutation
PML: Progressive Multifocal Leukoencephalopathy	TB: Tuberculosis
PrEP: Pre-Exposure Prophylaxis	TDM: Therapeutic Drug Monitoring
PI/c: Cobicistat-boosted Protease Inhibitor	TEN: Toxic Epidermal Necrolysis
PI/r: RTV boosted Protease Inhibitor	tid: three times per day
PML: Progressive Multifocal Leukoencephalopathy	tiw: three times per week
PMTCT: Prevention of Mother-To-Child Transmission	TMP/SMX: Trimethoprim + sulfamethoxazole
po: by mouth	ULN: Upper Limit of Normal
q: every	VL: Viral Load
qd: daily	VZIG: Varicella Zoster Immune Globulin
qid: four times per day	VZV: Varicella Zoster Virus
qm: monthly	X4-tropic Virus: HIV strains that enter the CD4 cell using the CXCR4 coreceptor

FORMULAS

TABLE 3A: **Child-Pugh Score (CPS) for Hepatic Disease**

Component	1 point	2 points	3 points
Encephalopathy	None	Gr 1-2	Gr 3-4
Ascites	None	Mild	Mod/Refractory
Albumin (g/dL)	> 3.5	2.8-3.5	< 2.8
Total bilirubin (mg/dL)	< 2	2-3	> 3
Pro-time sec. or INR	< 4 < 1.7	4-6 1.7-2.3	> 6 > 2.3

CP Classification
5-6 points: C-P A
7-9 points: C-P B
> 9 points: C-P C

Encephalopathy score
Gr 1: Mild confusion, fine tremor
Gr 2: Confusion, asterixis, disoriented
Gr 3: Somnolent, incontinence, imcomprehensible
Gr 4: Coma, decerebrate posture, flaccid

TABLE 3B: **Creatinine Clearance**

Males:	$\frac{\text{Weight (kg) x (140-age)}}{\text{72 x Serum creatinine (mg/dL)}}$
Females:	*Value for males x 0.85*
Note: Assumes stable renal function.	

TABLE 4: **CDC HIV Staging System** (*MMWR* 2014; 63 (RK03:1-10)

Stage	CD4	CD4%	Clinical
1	> 500	≥ 26%	No AIDS-defining dx
2	200-499	14-25%	No AIDS-defining dx
3	< 200	< 14%	AIDS-defining dx

TABLE 5: **AIDS-defining diagnoses**

Definitions and frequency with CDC reported data for 1997 based on 23,527 US cases (last year the CDC collected and reported these data).

Candidiasis – esophagus, trachea, lungs – 16%

Cervical cancer, invasive – 0.6%

Coccidioidomycosis, extrapulmonary – 0.3%

Cryptococcosis, extrapulmonary – 5.0%

Cryptosporidiosis with diarrhea > 1 month – 1.3%

CMV – any organ but the liver, spleen, nodes (eye) – 7%

HSV with mucocutaneous ulcer > 1 month or bronchitis, pneumonia, esophagitis – 5%

Histoplasmosis, extrapulmonary – 0.9%

HIV dementia – disabling cognitive or other dysfunction interfering with normal function – 5%

Isosporoiasis with diarrhea > 1 month – 0.1%

Kaposi sarcoma – 7%

Lymphoma

- Burkitt – 0.7%
- immunoblastic – 2.3%
- primary CNS – 0.7%

M. avium or ***M. kansasii*** infection – extrapulmonary 5%

Tuberculosis

- pulmonary – 7%
- extrapulmonary – 2%

Pneumocystis **pneumonia** – 38%

Pneumonia, recurrent bacterial with > 2 episodes in 12 months – 5%

Progressive multifocal leukoencephalophy – 1%

Salmonellosis (nontyphoid), recurrent – 0.3%

Toxoplasmosis – internal organ – 4%

BASELINE EVALUATION

TABLE 6: **Laboratory Tests**

(DHHS ART Guidelines 2016; IDSA/HIVMA Primary Care Guidelines: *Aberg J CID 2014; 58:1*)

Test	Comment
HIV screening test	• 4th generation test (p24 Ag and HIV Ab) now preferred to detect early infection p24Ag and HIV antibody for HIV-1 and HIV-2. HIV testing algorithm (http://stacks.cdc.gov/view/cdc/23446). • Sensitivity and specificity standard serology is > 99% False positives: Usually human error False negatives: Usually 'window period' (uncommon with 4th gen test)
CD4 count and %	• Reproducibility: 95% CI: 30% • False high levels - splenectomy (use CD4%) or concurrent HTLV-1 (serologic test) • Repeat q3-6 mos; prior to ART, and during first 2 years of ART, during viremia, if receiving ART or if CD4 < 300/mm^3 • Repeat q12 month if on ART ≥ 2 years with viral suppression and CD4 300-500/mm^3. • CD8 count and CD4/CD8 ratio are unnecessary and increase costs of test. • CD4 monitoring optional if on ART ≥ 2 years with viral suppression and
HIV viral load	• Test at diagnosis; before starting ART; q2-4 weeks after initiating ART; thereafter q4-8 weeks until VL undetectable; within 2-4 after virologic failure; q3-4 months during the first 2 years of ART, q6 month after 2 years of ART with consistent VL suppression. • Reproducibility: 95% CI - 0.3 $\log_{10}$ c/mL or 50%
Genotypic Resistance Test	• Genotypic resistance test at diagnosis and with virologic failure while on ART or within 4 wks of stopping ART. • Test at initiation of ART in pregnant women; optional in others if resistance genotype done at diagnosis.
CBC	• Repeat every 3-6 mos; more frequently as indicated (AZT) and co-morbidities • Repeat with treatment initiation or change. • Macrocytosis with AZT and d4T
Chemistry Profile (Creatinine, BUN, ALT, AST, Alk phos)	• Baseline, at initiation of ART; repeat q6-12 mo • Repeat LFT q3-6 mos on ART and as clinically indicated • Repeat renal function with IDV & TDF (and possibly ATV and cobicistat) q3-6 mos
Hepatitis Screen: Anti-HAV, Anti-HCV, Anti-HBsAg, Anti-HBcAg, and HBsAg	• Standard screen: anti-HCV, anti-HAV, HBsAg, HBsAb, and anti-HBc • Abnormal LFT: anti-HCV & HBsAg • Neg anti-HCV: not infected. Check HCV VL in pts at risk (e.g. IVDU) • Positive anti-HCV only: quantitative HCV RNA and HCV genotype • Positive HBsAg indicates acute or chronic: order HBV DNA, antiHBc, HBeAg • If HBsAg pos at baseline: treat HIV and HBV using TDF/FTC or TDF+3TC as NRTI backbone. • If anti-HBc positive but HBsAb negative, order HBV DNA. If negative, vaccinate • If HBsAg and HBsAb are negative: give HBV vaccine • Negative anti-HAV: HAV vaccine if risks (MSM, IDU, travelers) or consider in all non-immune pts;; Positive anti-HAV: immune
Fasting lipid Profile:	• Assess cardiovascular risk. Test lipids at entry to care, at initiation of ART, then annually if normal or 4-8 weeks after starting or changing ART that affects lipids, then q6 mo if abnormal last test or if clinically indicated.
FBS and Hgb A1c	• FBS: Entry to care, prior to ART, q3-6 mo if last test abnormal or annually.

(continued)

TABLE 6: **Laboratory Tests** *(cont.)*

Test	Comment
Toxoplasma IgG	• 10-30% positive in US; 50-80% in developing countries • If negative repeat if suspicion of toxoplasmosis (cannot be used to confirm or exclude Dx) or when CD4< 100/mm³
PPD or Interferon Gamma Release Assay (IGRA)	• IGRA advantages: more specific, one clinic visit, no BCG false positive, but increased cost. • Indicated if no history of TB or prior positive PPD • May be false negative with HIV • Induration > 5 mm or + IGRA is indication latent or possibly active TB treatment. In patients at low risk for LTBI, consider repeat testing before latent TB treatment. • Chest X-ray to r/o active TB before latent TB treatment
Pap smear	• Baseline, at 6 mos, and then annual; if 'inadequate' repeat; if atypia - refer to gynecologist • HIVMA/IDSA HIV Primary care guidelines and Cytology ("anal pap smears") for at risk MSM (anal receptive intercourse) and women with history of anal sex or abnormal cervical Paps.
Urinary NAAT for *N. gonorrhoeae*, *Chlamydia trachomatis* and Trichomoniasis	• All women should be screened for trichomoniasis • Women < 25 yrs should be screened for *C. trachomatis* • Consider: in sexually active patients (see Table 53) • Repeat at 6-12 mos intervals depending on risk
HLA B*5701	• Screening before ABC treatment; negative test virtually excludes risk of ABC hypersensitivity reaction
Tropism Assay	• Screening before use of MVC. • Phenotypic *Trofile* is more expensive than newer genotypic assays. • R-5-tropic virus present in approximately 80% of treatment-naive patients vs. 40-60% in treatment-experienced.
Direct Treponemal Enzyme Immunoassay, then reflex to Non-treponemal tests (RPR)	• False positive RPR and low sensitivity in early primary and treated infections • Due to the ability to automate Treponemal EIAs and reduce lab cost, direct Treponemal test is done first, followed by confirmation with RPR. • Positive EIA with negative RPR, requires confirmation with Treponema pallidum particle agglutination (TP-PA)
Renal Screen (urinalysis, Scr)	• Urinalysis and creatinine; entry to care, initiation of ART, repeat annually, q6 mo if underlying renal disease or on TDF. • If > 1+ proteinuria or elevated creatinine: quantify urine protein and order renal ultrasound if HIVAN suspected
G6PD Level	• Consider: most susceptible are men of African, Mediterranean, Asian, or Sephardic Jewish descent. Rate in African-American -10%, Hispanics - 2%, Caucasians - 0.7% (JID 2010;61:399) • If pos, avoid oxidant drugs dapsone and primaquine; ? sulfonamides. Rate of significant hemolysis with positive G6PD + TMP/SMX reported at 7% (*JID* 2010;61:399)

(continued)

TABLE 6: **Laboratory Tests** *(cont.)*

Test	Comment
Chest X-Ray	• Recommended for patients with pulmonary symptoms, history of a chronic chest disease or positive screening test for TB
CMV IgG; VZV IgG	• Identifies chronic infection. • Diagnostic: Consider CMV IgG in patients at low risk for CMV • VZV IgG recommended in those who don't recall history of chickenpox or shingles.
Testosterone	• Consider in men with fatigue, weight loss, decreased libido, erectile dysfunction, depression or osteoporosis • Obtain morning free serum testosterone
General Health Screens (Recommendations of US Public Service Task Force)	
Mammography	Biennial for women 50-74 yrs; optional age 40-49 (USPSTF2015)
Prostate Specific Antigen (PSA)	Recommended by American Cancer Society, but not USPSTF. Discuss pros and cons with patient.
Colorectal Cancer screening	Test occult blood, sigmoidoscopy, or colonoscopy age 50-75 years (USPSTF 2008)
Bone Densitometry	Recommended based on osteoporosis or FRAX score • National Osteoporosis Foundation: Women > 65 yrs, fragility fracture or persons > 50 yrs with risk (not including HIV) • HIVMA/IDSA HIV Primary Care Guildelines (*CID* 2014; 58:1): All HIV positive post-menopausal women and men > 50 yrs and all with fragility fractures

TABLE 7: **Laboratory Monitoring Before and During ART**

(DHHS Guidelines 2016)*

Test	Baseline	Before ART	ART Initiation	wk 2-8 follow-up	Every 3-6 Mo	Every 6-12 Mo	Viral Failure or clinically indicated
CD4	+	q3-6 mos	+		+ (first 2 years of ART; viremia on ART; CD4<300)	+ After 2 years of ART with VL <50 with CD4 300-500 q12 mos; Optional if VL < 50 and CD4 >500	+
Viral Load	+	optional	+	If VL >200	If VL <200	Every 6 months	+
Genotypic Resistance Test	+		+				+
Hepatitis B serology	+		+ (if neg at baseline)				+
Basic Chemistry	+	q6-12 mos	+	+	+		+
AST, ALT, Total Bilirubin	+	q6-12 mos	+	+	+		+

* Repeat testing if clinically indicated

TABLE 7: Laboratory Monitoring Before and During ART (cont.)

Test	Baseline	Before ART	ART Initiation	wk 2-8 follow-up	Every 3-6 Mo	Every 6-12 Mo	Viral Failure or clinically indicated
CBC	+	q3-6 mos	+	+ (AZT)	+		+
Lipids/ FBS or A1C	+	Annual	+	*	*	+	+
Urinalysis	+		+		q6 mos with TDF	+	+

* Repeat testing if clinically indicated

TABLE 8: CD4 Cell Count Correlation between CD4 count and CD4%:

CD4 Count	CD4%
> 500 cells/mm^3	> 28%
200-500 cells/mm^3	14-28%
< 200 cells/mm^3	< 14%

Normal levels: 800-1050 cells/mm^3 (95% CI=500-1400 cells/mm^3)

Reproducibility: Approximately 30% for 2 SD; thus, a CD4 count of 200 could be reported at 118-337 cells/mm^3

Deceptively high counts: Splenectomy or HTLV-1 infection

CD4%: Less variable metric

Recommendations for CD4 count testing (DHHS 2016): Entry to care, q3-6 months prior to ART, q3-6 months first 2 years of ART, or if viremia during ART or if CD4 count <200; With VL suppression on ART and CD4 300-500: q12 months; CD4 > 500 and VL suppression: CD4 count monitoring is optional.

Expected CD4 response to ART:

Time	cells/mm^3
4-8 weeks	+50
1 year	+100-150
5 years	+20-50/year

TABLE 9: Viral Load

Reproducibility: 2 SD = 3-fold or 0.5 $\log_{10}$ c/mL; thus, 95% CI for a VL of 10,000 c/mL would be 3,100-32,000 c/mL

Recommendations for Viral Load testing (DHHS Guidelines 2016): Entry to care; initiation of ART; if HIV RNA detectable at 2-8 weeks, repeat q4-8 wks until VL <200, then q3-6 months

Expected VL response to ART:

Treatment	VL ($\log_{10}$/mL)*
1 week	Decrease 0.75-1.0
4 weeks	Decrease 1.5-2.0; <5000 c/mL
8-16 weeks	< 500 c/mL
24-48 weeks	< 20 c/mL

* more rapid virologic response observed with InSTI-based regimens

TABLE 10: **ARV formulations, dosing, and ADRs**

Formulations(s)	Brand	Pill	Usual adult dose	Adverse Events
Once-Daily Co-Formulated ARV Regimens				
Dolutegravir/ abacavir/ lamivudine* (DTG/ABC/3TC) 50/600/300 mg tablet	Triumeq	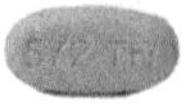	One tablet once-daily with or without food.	-Generally well tolerated in clinical trials with less discontinuation than with comparator ARVs (EFV, DRV/r) -DTG hypersensitivity reaction including rash, constitutional symptoms, and liver injury (rare). -Abacavir hypersensitivity reaction in HLA B*5701 positive pts (must pre-screen with HLA B*5701). -Possible HBV flare with 3TC discontinuation -Insomnia; headache -CK elevation -DTG: Serum creatinine elevation (no change in true GFR) -ABC: Possible increased risk of MI (controversial)
Efavirenz/ tenofovir DF*/ emtricitabine* (EFV/TDF/FTC) 600/300/200 mg tablet	Atripla	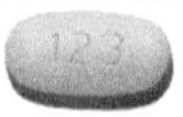	One tablet qhs without food. Can be taken with food or in the morning if tolerated	-EFV: Morbilliform rash in up to 26% of pts requiring discontinuation in 1.7% (median onset 11 days, duration 16 days) -EFV: Teratogenic in non-human primates, but can be used in pregnant patients after 8 week gestation -EFV: CNS side effects: vivid dreams including nightmares, nocturnal dizziness, morning confusion; depersonalization, possible suicidality (worse during the first 2 weeks, but can persist) -EFV: False positive THC and benzodiazepine screening test -EFV: Hyperlipidemia -EFV: Increased LFTs -TDF: nephrotoxicity -TDF: early loss of bone density -TDF/FTC: Possible HBV flare with discontinuation
Elvitegravir/ cobicistat/ tenofovir alafenamide*/ emtricitabine* (EVG/COBI/TAF /FTC) 150/150/10/ 200 mg tablet	Genvoya	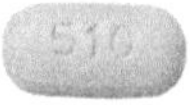	One tablet once-daily with food.	Generally well tolerated TAF: lower rates of nephrotoxicity than TDF, but do not use with CrCL <30 ml/min GI intolerance: nausea, diarrhea TAF/FTC: possible HBV flare with discontinuation TAF: lower rates of BMD loss than TDF FTC: skin hyperpigmentation
Elvitegravir/ cobicistat/ tenofovir DF*/ emtricitabine* (EVG/COBI/TDF/ FTC) 150/150/300/ 200 mg tablet	Stribild	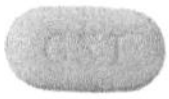	One tablet once-daily with food.	-Generally well tolerated with numerically lower discontinuation rates compared to EFV/TDF/FTC and ATV/r + TDF/FTC -TDF: nephrotoxicity (avoid in pts with CrCL <70 ml/min)-COBI: Serum creatinine elevation (no change in true GFR) -GI intolerance: nausea, diarrhea -TDF/FTC: Possible HBV flare with discontinuation -TDF: early loss of bone density -FTC: Skin hyperpigmentation.

*See Table 60 for dosing in renal failure

TABLE 10: **ARV formulations, dosing, and ADRs** *(cont.)*

Once-Daily Co-Formulated ARV Regimens				
Rilpivirine/ tenofovir alafenamide*/ emtricitabine* (RPV/TAF/FTC) 25/25/200 mg tablet	Odefsey	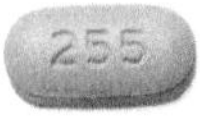	One tablet once-daily with food.	-Poorer performance with VL >100K and CD4 <200 -RPV: dose dependent QTc prolongation; monitor QTc with PI/r, COBI, and other CYP3A4 inhibitors -TAF: lower rates of nephrotoxicity than TDF, but do not use with CrCL <30 ml/min -GI intolerance: nausea, diarrhea -TAF/FTC: possible HBV flare with discontinuation -TAF: lower rates of BMD loss than TDF -FTC: skin hyperpigmentation
Rilpivirine/ tenofovir DF*/ emtricitabine* (RPV/TDF/FTC) 25/300/200 mg tablet	Complera	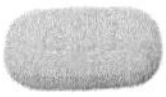	One tablet once-daily with food.	-Better tolerated than EFV/TDF/FTC -Poorer performance with VL >100K and CD4 <200 -TDF: nephrotoxicity -TDF: early loss of bone density -TDF/FTC: Possible HBV flare with discontinuation -RPV: Dose dependent QTc prolongation; monitor QTc closely with PI/r, COBI, and other CYP3A inhibitors. -RPV: Absorption dependent on food and gastric acid; must be taken with meal, and not with PPIs -RPV: resistance with 138K mutation leads to etravirine cross-resistance
Co-Formulated nucleoside reverse transcriptase inhibitors (NRTIs)				
Abacavir/ lamivudine* (ABC/3TC) 600/300mg tablet	Epzicom	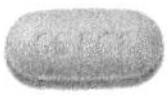	One tablet once-daily with or without food.	-Inferior VL response with VL >100K when combined with EFV or ATV/r, but not with DTG -ABC hypersensitivity reaction in HLA B*5701 positive pts (must prescreen with HLA B*5701). -ABC: Possible increased risk of MI (controversial) -TDF/FTC: Possible HBV flare with discontinuation
Zidovudine*/ abacavir/ lamivudine* (AZT/ABC/3TC) 300/300/150 mg tablet	Trizivir	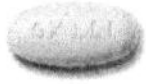	One tablet twice-daily with or without food.	-ABC hypersensitivity reaction in HLA B*5701 positive pts (must pre-screen with HLA B*5701). -AZT: GI intolerance: nausea, vomiting -AZT: Headache, asthenia -AZT: Bone marrow suppression (macrocytic anemia, neutropenia) -AZT: Mitochondrial toxicity with (lactic acidosis, hepatic steatosis)-must discontinue -AZT: Lipoatrophy, myopathy -ABC: Possible increased risk of MI (controversial) -3TC: Possible HBV flare with 3TC discontinuation

*See Table 60 for dosing in renal failure

TABLE 10: **ARV formulations, dosing, and ADRs** *(cont.)*

Co-Formulated nucleoside reverse transcriptase inhibitors (NRTIs)				
Tenofovir alafenamide* /emtricitabine* (TAF/FTC) 25/200 mg tablet	Descovy		One tablet once-daily with or without food	-Generally well tolerated -Lower rates of nephrotoxicity than TDF -Lower rates of BMD Loss than TDF -GI intolerance and nausea -Possible HBV flare with TAF/FTC discontinuation
Tenofovir*/ emtricitabine* (TDF/FTC) 300/200 mg tablet	Truvada		One tablet once-daily with or without food	-Generally well tolerated -TDF: GI intolerance: nausea, vomiting, diarrhea, flatulence -TDF: Nephrotoxicity, including proximal tubular dysfunction -TDF/FTC: Possible HBV flare with TDF/FTC discontinuation -TDF: Early loss of bone density. -TDF: Headache
Zidovudine•/ lamivudine• (AZT/3TC) 300/150 mg tablet	Combivir		One tablet twice-daily with or without food.	-AZT: GI intolerance: nausea, vomiting -AZT: Headache, asthenia -AZT: Bone marrow suppression (macrocytic anemia, neutropenia) -AZT: Mitochondrial toxicity (Lactic acidosis, hepatic steatosis)-must discontinue -AZT: Lipoatrophy, myopathy -AZT: Nail hyperpigmentation-3TC -Possible HBV flare with 3TC discontinuation
Co-formulated boosted Protease Inhibitors (PI/cobi)				
Atazanavir/ cobicistat (ATV/c) 300/150 mg Tablet	Evotaz	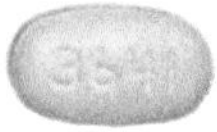	One tablet once-daily with food	-GI intolerance: nausea, vomiting, diarrhea -LFT elevation -ATV: Benign increase in indirect bilirubin, but may cause jaundice and/or scleral icterus -PR interval prolongation -COBI: Increase in serum creatine (no change in actual GFR) -ATV: Nephrotoxicity with or without nephrolithiasis (reported with ATV/r) -ATV: Cholelithiasis -Rash
Darunavir/ cobicistat (DRV/c) 800/150 mg tablet	Precobix		One tablet once-daily with food	-GI intolerance: nausea, vomiting, diarrhea -Rash (contains a sulfonamide moiety, but not contraindicated with sulfa allergy). Avoid with a history of severe sulfa allergy (eg SJS/TEN) -COBI: increase serum creatinine (no change in actual GFR). -Hepatitis -Headache
Nucleoside reverse transcriptase inhibitors (NRTIs)				
Abacavir (ABC) 300 mg tablet 20 mg/ml solution	Ziagen, generic	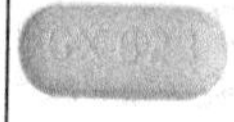	600mg once-daily with or without food	-ABC hypersensitivity reaction in HLA B*5701 positive pts (must pre-screen with HLA B*5701). -Possible increased risk of MI (controversial) -Less effective at VL >100,000 when combined with EFV or ATV/r, but not DTG

*See Table 60 for dosing in renal failure

TABLE 10: **ARV formulations, dosing, and ADRs** *(cont.)*

Nucleoside reverse transcriptase inhibitors (NRTIs)				
Didanosine* (ddI) 125, 200, 250, 400 mg EC capsules 10 mg/mL solution	Videx. generic		>60kg: 400 mg once-daily <60kg: 250 mg once-daily With TDF co-administration: ddI 250 mg once-daily	-Mitochondrial toxicity (lactic acidosis, hepatic steatosis peripheral neuropathy and pancreatitis)-must discontinue -GI intolerance: nausea, vomiting -Possible increase in MI risk -Insulin resistance/DM -Possible non-cirrhotic portal -Not recommended
Emtricitabine* (FTC) 200 mg gel capsule 10 mg/mL solution	Emtriva	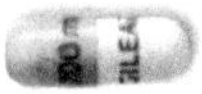	200mg once-daily	-Generally well tolerated -Possible HBV flare with discontinuation -Skin hyperpigmentation
Lamivudine* (3TC) 150 mg and 300 mg tablets 10 mg/mL oral solution	Epivir, generic	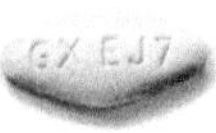	300mg once daily or 150 mg twice-daily	-Generally well tolerated -Possible HBV flare in co-infected pts with 3TC discontinuation
Stavudine* (d4T) 15, 20,30, and 40 mg capsules 1mg/ml oral solution	Zerit, generic	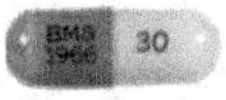	40 mg twice daily (but associated with greater toxicity) 30 mg twice-daily	-Mitochondrial toxicity (lactic acidosis, hepatic steatosis peripheral neuropathy)-must discontinue -Lipoatrophy -Progressive ascending neuromuscular weakness (rare)-must discontinue -Insulin resistance/DM -Hyperlipidemia -Not recommended
Tenofovir* (TDF) 150, 200, 250, 300 mg tablets 40 mg/g oral powder	Viread	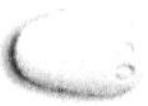	300 mg once-daily with or without food.	-Generally well tolerated -GI intolerance: nausea, vomiting, diarrhea, flatulence -Nephrotoxicity, including proximal tubular dysfunction -Early decrease in bone density -Possible HBV flare with discontinuation -Potential decrease in BMD. -Headache
Zidovudine* (AZT) 100 mg capsule and 300 mg tablet 10 mg/mL oral solution 10mg/mL IV solution	Retrovir, generic	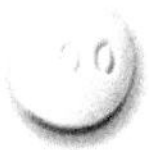	300 mg twice-daily with or without food.	-GI intolerance: nausea, vomiting -Headache, asthenia -Bone marrow suppression (macrocytic anemia, neutropenia) -Mitochondrial toxicity (lactic acidosis, hepatic steatosis)-must discontinue -Lipoatrophy -Myopathy -Nail hyperpigmentation

*See Table 60 for dosing in renal failure

TABLE 10: **ARV formulations, dosing, and ADRs** *(cont.)*

Non-nucleoside reverse transcriptase inhibitors (NNRTIs)				
Efavirenz (EFV) 600mg tablet 50 mg and 200mg capsules	Sustiva	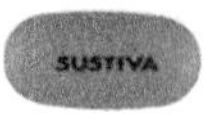	600mg once qhs on an empty stomach.	-Morbilliform rash in up to 26% of pts requiring discontinuation in 1.7% -Teratogenic in non-human primates, but can be used in pregnant patients after 8 weeks -CNS side effects: vivid dreams including nightmares, nocturnal dizziness, morning confusion; depersonalization, and possible suicidality (worse during the first 2 weeks, but may persist) -False positive THC and benzodiazepine screening test -Hyperlipidemia -Increased LFTs
Etravirine (ETR) 25, 100 and 200mg tablets	Intelence		200mg twice daily with food. 400 mg once daily may be considered based on PK studies.	-Generally well tolerated -GI: nausea -Rash: generally mild to moderate (but SJS has been reported), occurs in 2nd wk and resolves within 1-2 wks on continued therapy. SJS has been reported. -HSR reaction: Rash, constitutional Sx, hepatitis; discontinue ETR.
Nevirapine (NVP) 200 mg tablet and 400mg XR tablet 50mg/5mL oral suspension	Viramune, generic	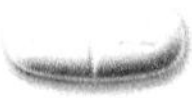	200 mg once daily x 2 wks then 200mg twice daily (OR 400 mg XR tab once daily) with or without food. Avoid initiating in men with pre-treatment CD4 >400 men women with CD4 >250.	-Rash is common (up to 50% of pts). Severe rashes including SJS and TEN more common compared to other NNRTIs -Severe hepatitis, including fatal hepatic necrosis (increased risk win women with CD4 >250 and men with CD4 >400 at initiation of therapy).
Rilpivirine (RPV) 25mg tablet	Edurant		25mg once daily with food. Food and acidic gastric pH critical for absorption. Avoid antacids, H2-blockers, PPIs	-Hepatitis -Dose dependent QTc prolongation -Depression (8%; most were mild or moderate in severity. The rate of Grade 3 or 4 depression was 1%) -Insomnia, headache
Protease Inhibitors (PIs)				
Atazanavir (ATV) 100, 150, 200, and 300 mg capsules	Reyataz		400 mg once daily OR 300 mg (plus ritonavir 100 mg or cobicistat 150 mg) once daily with food With EFV, use ATV 400 mg + RTV 100 mg. Avoid antacid, H-2 blocker, and PPIs or use with recommended dose separation.	-GI intolerance: nausea, vomiting, diarrhea -Hyperlipidemia with boosted ATV, but less common compared to older PIs. -Benign increase in indirect bilirubin; may cause jaundice or scleral icterus -PR interval prolongation including first degree block -Nephrotoxicity with or without nephrolithiasis -Cholelithiasis -Rash

*See Table 60 for dosing in renal failure

TABLE 10: **ARV formulations, dosing, and ADRs** *(cont.)*

Protease Inhibitors (PIs)				
Darunavir (DRV) 75, 150, 600 and 800mg tablets 100 mg/mL oral suspension	Prezista	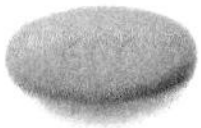	800mg with ritonavir 100mg <u>or</u> cobicistat 150 mg once daily OR 600mg with ritonavir 100mg twice daily with food. Twice-daily dosing recommended in pts with DRV-associated mutations.	-GI intolerance: nausea, vomiting, diarrhea -Rash reported in 10% (contains a sulfonamide moiety, but not contraindicated in patents with sulfa allergy). Avoid with a history of severe sulfa allergy (eg JS/TEN) -Hepatitis -Headache
Fosamprenavir (FPV) 700mg tablet 50 mg/mL oral suspension	Lexiva	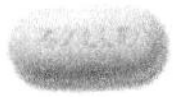	FPV/r 700/100 mg twice daily OR FPV/r 1400 /100 mg once daily (PI-naïve only) with or without food. FPV 1400 mg twice-daily (not recommended) With EFV co-administration, FPV/r 1400/300 mg once-daily OR FPV/r 700/100 mg twice-daily.	-GI intolerance: nausea, vomiting, diarrhea -Rash reported in 12-19% (contains a sulfonamide moiety). Avoid with a history of severe sulfa allergy (eg SJS/TEN) -Hepatitis -Headache -Nephrolithiasis (rare) -May increase risk of bleed in pts with hemophilia -Resistance (usually with unboosted FPV) can lead to DRV-cross-resistance -Not a recommended PI (DHHS guidelines)
Indinavir (IDV) 100, 200, 400 mg capsules	Crixivan	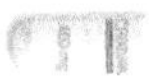	IDV 800 mg q8h 1 hr or 2 hrs after meals. IDV/r 800/100 mg twice-daily	-PI class ADR: Hyperglycemia, LFTs elevation, fat accumulation, hyperlipidemia -Asthenia, headache, metallic taste -GI intolerance: nausea, vomiting, diarrhea -Benign increase in indirect bilirubin; may cause jaundice or scleral icterus -May increase risk of bleed in pts with hemophilia -Nephrolithiasis, nephrotoxicity -Retinoid effects: paronychia, xerosis, hair loss
Lopinavir/ritonavir (LPV/r) 200/50 mg mg Tablet 400/100 mg per 5 ml oral solution	Kaletra	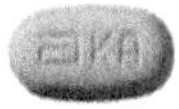	LPV/r 400/100 twice daily OR LPV/r 800/200 mg once daily with or without food	-PI class ADR: Hyperglycemia, LFTs elevation, fat accumulation, hyperlipidemia -GI intolerance: nausea, vomiting, diarrhea (higher rates than ATV/r and DRV/r). -QTc and PR prolongation -May increase risk of bleed in pts with hemophilia -Asthenia -Pancreatitis
Nelfinavir (NFV) 250 mg and 625 mg tablets 50mg/g oral powder	Viracept	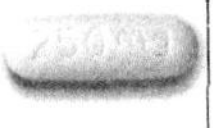	NFV 1250 mg twice daily with fatty meals OR NFV 750 mg three times a day with fatty meals.	-PI class ADR: Hyperglycemia, LFTs elevation, fat accumulation, hyperlipidemia -GI intolerance: nausea, vomiting, secretory diarrhea -May increase risk of bleed in pts with hemophilia -Inferior virologic suppression compared to other PIs and cannot be boosted: Not recommended

*See Table 60 for dosing in renal failure

TABLE 10: **ARV formulations, dosing, and ADRs** *(cont.)*

Protease Inhibitors (PIs)				
Saquinavir (SQV) 500 mg and 200 mg capsule	Invirase	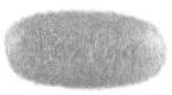	SQV/r 1000/100 mg twice-daily.	-PI class ADR: Hyperglycemia, LFTs elevation, fat accumulation, hyperlipidemia -GI intolerance: nausea, vomiting, diarrhea -Hepatitis -QTc (avoid if QTc >450 ms) -PR prolongation -May increase risk of bleed in pts with hemophilia
Tipranavir (TPV) 250mg capsulte 100 mg/mL oral solution	Aptivus	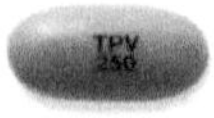	TPV/r 500/200mg twice-daily with food.	-PI class ADR: Hyperglycemia, LFTs elevation, fat accumulation, hyperlipidemia -GI intolerance: nausea, vomiting, diarrhea -Rash reported in 3-21% (contains a sulfonamide moiety). Avoid with a history of severe sulfa allergy (eg SJS/TEN) -May increase risk of bleed in pts with hemophilia -High incidence of hepatitis including fatalities -Intracranial hemorrhage (rare) -Recommended only for use in treatment experienced patients with virus that is resistant to other PIs but susceptible to TPV
Integrase Inhibitors (INSTI)				
Dolutegravir (DTG) 50mg tablet	Tivicay		50mg once-daily with or without food <u>or</u> 50 mg twice-daily with or without food if integrase mutations present. 50 mg twice-daily when combined with FPV/r, TPV/r, EFV.	-Generally well tolerated in clinical trials with more patients discontinuing comparator ARVs (EFV, DRV/r) -DTG hypersensitivity reaction including rash, constitutional symptoms, and liver injury (rare). -Insomnia, headache -CK elevation -Serum creatinine elevation without change in actual GFR
Elvitegravir (EVG) 85 mg and 150mg tablet	Vitekta	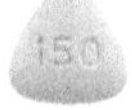	With ATV/r 300/100 mg once-daily or LPV/r 400/100 mg twice daily: EVG 85mg once-daily with food With DRV/r 600/100 mg, FPV/r 700/100 mg, or TPV/r 500/200 mg twice-daily: EVG 150 mg once daily with food	-Generally well tolerated -Gi Intolerance: Diarrhea; diarrhea -See page 23 for ADR of pharmacokinetic enhancer (COBI and RTV)
Raltegravir (RAL) 400mg tablet 25 and 100 mg chewable tablets 100 mg per pack oral suspension	Isentress	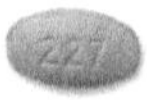	400mg twice-daily with or without food.	-Generally well tolerated in clinical trials, with comparable ADR rates to placebo in clinical trials. -GI intolerance: nausea, diarrhea -CK elevation (rhabdomyolysis reported) -Headache, insomnia -Fever (unclear association) -Rash (rare cases of SJS, HSR, and TEN reported)

*See Table 60 for dosing in renal failure

TABLE 10: ARV formulations, dosing, and ADRs (cont.)

Entry Inhibitors (fusion inhibitor and CCR5 blocker)				
Enfuvirtide (T20) 90 mg/mL vial	Fuzeon	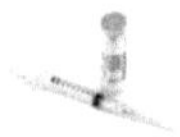	90 mg (1mL) SC twice-daily	-Injection site reaction (e.g pain, erythema, induration) -Rare cases of hypersensitivity reaction (rash, fever, chills, hepatitis, nausea, vomiting, and hypotension)-Do not rechallenge. -Possible increased risk of bacterial pneumonia
Maraviroc* (MVC) 150 and 300mg tablets	Selzentry		-With all NRTIs, DTG, RAL, TPV/r, RPV (without PIs, COBI, EFV, or ETR): MVC 300 mg twice-daily -With all PIs (except TPV/r) and COBI: MVC 150 mg twice-daily. -With EFV and ETR (without a PI): MVC 600 mg twice daily If RTV- or COBI-boosted regimen given with EFV or ETR: MVC 150 mg twice-daily. Must pre-screen for R5 tropism	-Generally well tolerated in clinical trials, with similar rates of discontinuation vs. placebo -GI: diarrhea, nausea, abdominal pain -CK elevation, myalgia -Hepatotoxicity (preceded by severe rash and eosinophilia, elevated IgE) -Fever -Dizziness
Pharmacokinetic Enhancer/CYP3A4 inhibitor				
Cobicistat (COBI or /c) 150 mg tablet	Tybost		150 mg once daily with food in combination with DRV 800 mg once-daily OR ATV 300 mg once-daily	-GI intolerance -Increased serum creatinine without effect on actual GFR
Ritonavir (RTV) 100mg tablet 100 mg soft gel capsule 80mg/mL oral solution	Norvir		Pharmacoenhancer (booster) of other PIs: 100 – 200mg once or twice a day FDA labeled full dose of 600 mg twice a day: not recommended.	-PI class ADR: Hyperglycemia, LFTs elevation, fat accumulation, hyperlipidemia -Dose dependent GI intolerance: nausea, vomiting, diarrhea -Dose dependent hepatitis -Circumoral paresthesia, asthenia, taste perversion associated with full dose RTV.

TABLE 11: Adverse Reactions of Antiretroviral Agents

Life Threatening Reactions	
Hepatic Necrosis	
Agent	NVP
ADR Features	Abrupt onset of flu-like illness with GI symptoms, fever, rash (50%), eosinophilia and hepatic necrosis usually in first 6 wks and up to 18 weeks.
Frequency	1-2% of all NVP recipients. Rate of symptomatic hepatitis is 11% in treatment-naive women with baseline CD4 count > 250 cells/mm^3 and 6% in men with baseline CD4 count > 400 cells/mm^3. No risk with single dose for PMTCT.
Monitor	Warn patient. ALT: Baseline and at 2 wks and 4 wks; then monthly x 3 mos, then q3mos.
Intervention	Promptly discontinue ART, but may progress despite this. Supportive care (steroids, antihistamines appear ineffective). Do not rechallenge Safety of NNRTI switch unknown.
Cutaneous: Stevens-Johnson Syndrome and Toxic Epidermal Necrolysis	
Agent	NVP; less common with EFV, ETR, RPV (reported with FPV, DRV, TPV, ABC, ddI, LPV, AZT, ATV, RAL and IDV).
ADR Features	Usually first few weeks with fever, myalgia, skin rash with blistering ± mucous membrane; involvement with NVP may also cause hepatic necrosis.
Frequency	NVP 0.5-1%, EFV 0.1%, ETR < 0.1%; RPV (uncommon)
Monitor	Warn patient
Intervention	Promptly discontinue ART if mucous membrane involved, conjunctivitis, blisters, bullae, and/or system symptoms. Intensive care of wounds including pain meds and antibiotics and IVs; may require treatment in a burn center. Role of steroids and IVIG unclear.
Lactic Acidosis	
Agent	d4T > ddI > AZT (Rare or never with ABC, TDF, 3TC, and FTC); more common w/ long duration use.
ADR Features	GI symptoms, wasting, fatigue, ± multiorgan failure, pancreatitis, respiratory failure.
Frequency	1-10 per 1,000 patient-years for d4T or ddI. Risk: d4T > ddI > AZT; Female, obesity; dose and duration related.
Monitor	Clinical symptoms. No routine lactate levels, but obtain if clinically indicated; normal level is < 2.0 mmol/L. Surrogate for lactic acid levels: High CPK and ALT; low HCO_3; anion gap.
Intervention	Promptly discontinue ART; supportive care with mechanical ventilation, dialysis, HCO_3 infusion, hemofiltration. Role of steroids, carnitine, thiamine, IVIG, plasmapheresis, or riboflavin: unclear. Recovery may take months. Long-term residual effects are common. For ART avoid NRTI or use ABC, 3TC, FTC, and/or TDF. Case reports of benefit from L-carnitine, riboflavin.

Life Threatening Reactions (cont.)	
Hypersensitivity (HSR)	
Agent	Common: ABC; NVP Uncommon: RAL (possibly DTG); MVC
ADR Features	ABC Symptoms (in rank order): high fever, diffuse skin rash, nausea, headache, abdominal pain, diarrhea, arthralgias, pharyngitis, and dyspnea. Virtually all have ≥ 2 systems involved (may help distinguish common intercurrent illnesses). Always progresses with continued ABC use. Median onset: day 9 of ABC; 90% in first 6 wks. NVP: see hepatic necrosis RAL: severe rash including rash w/ eosinophilia and systemic symptoms MVC: see hepatitis
Frequency	ABC: 6-7% of ABC recipients; very rare or never if HLA-B* 5701 is negative. Risk lower in African-Americans. NVP: Up to 11% in women with CDY $>$ 250
Monitor	ABC: Warn patient. (In questionable cases, administer next dose under observation - this reaction always progresses with next dose). NVP: Monitor for rash, hepatitis, fever in first 6-8 weeks
Intervention	ABC: D/C ABC. Never re-challenge (if dx is likely). Supportive care (steroids and antihistamines are not useful). Symptoms usually resolve in 48 h after D/C ABC. NVP: D/C NVP ASAP
Serious Reactions	
Pancreatitis	
Agent	ddI + d4T $>$ ddI $>$ d4T
ADR Features	Abdominal pain with elevated amylase and/or lipase.
Frequency	ddI 1-7%. More frequent with other risk factors-especially alcoholism, hx pancreatitis, concurrent d4T, ddI and TDF without ddI dose adjustment, ddI + ribavirin (contraindicated).
Monitor	Warn patient. Amylase and lipase with clinical symptoms.
Intervention	Supportive care, pain meds and bowel rest (NPO).
Nephrotoxicity	
Agent	TDF+boosted ATV>TDF>IDV>ATV (and possibly LPV/r)>TAF
ADR Features	TDF: Renal failure ± Proximal tubulopathy or full Fanconi syndrome. Note: increased creatinine, proteinuria, hypophosphotemia, renal phosphate wasting, glycosuria, hypokalemia, non-anion gap, metabolic acidosis. May be asymptomatic or signs of diabetes insipidus. Risks: Advanced age; low BMI, low CD4, concurrent use of PI/r or PI/c; avoid TDF with CrCl $<$ 50 mL/min unless end-stage renal disease. ATV/IDV: nephrotoxicity +/- nephrolithiasis
Frequency	Low, but increase with long term use and possibly with boosted PI co-administration.
Monitor	Monitor urinalysis and Scr. If proteinuria or decreased CrCL then measure urine protein/creatinine or albumin/creatinine ratio
Intervention	Evaluate and use alternative agent. Although not preferred, dose-adjusted TDF can be considered in selective cases if no evidence of tubulopathy.

TABLE 11: Adverse Reactions of Antiretroviral Agents

(con

Serious Reactions (cont.)	
Renal calculi	
Agent	IDV >> ATV
ADR Features	Renal colic, abdominal pain, hematuria. UA shows RBC, pyuria,and crystals.
Frequency	5-35%; correlates with high peak IDV blood level. ATV is uncommon cause
Monitor	Urinalysis ± creatinine or BUN q3-5mos with IDV.
Intervention	Avoid or D/C IDV. Prevention is hydration with ≥ 1.5 L/d with IDV. Manage as nephrolithiasis. IDV should be stopped or given with better hydration.
Bone marrow suppression	
Agent	ZDV
ADR Features	Neutropenia and/or anemia usually after weeks-months.
Frequency	Anemia 1-4%, neutropenia 2-8%. Risk increased with advanced HIV ANC < 500 in 2-8%.
Monitor	CBC at baseline and q3mos for ZDV recipients.
Intervention	Avoid or D/C AZT. Transfusion or EPO for serious anemia; GCSF for neutropenia. D/C ZDV.
Hepatitis	
Agent	All PIs (TPV/r>>all other PIs), NNRTIs, some NRTIs (d4T, ddI + AZT and MVC. Note: Discontinuation or development of resistance to 3TC, FTC, and TDF can cause HBV flare in HIV/HBV co-infection.
ADR Features	Elevated ALT that is otherwise not explained (ETOH, hepatitis B, hepatitis C etc). PI/NNRTI: mechanism is unknown. Liver biopsy usually does not show hepatic injury. Most are asymptomatic - exceptions are NVP-associated hepatic necrosis and NRTI-associated lactic acidosis (AZT, d4T, ddI) with steatosis. MVC hepatitis preceded by rash and increased IgE. ddI: non-cirrhotic portal hypertension
Frequency	8-15% for most PIs and NNRTIs.
Monitor	ALT q3-4mos
Intervention	Must distinguish ALT elevations due to other drugs (lactic acidosis with steatosis due to d4T, ddI or ZDV), from hypersensitivity due to ABC, or NVP hepatic necrosis) and other causes (hepatitis viruses, IRIS, ETOH, etc). Many D/C the PI or NNRTI if the ALT is > 5x ULN (Grade 3 toxicity) or 10x ULN (Grade 4), or if symptomatic or ↑ Bilirubin (Total) > 2x ULN with ALT > 3x ULN.

TABLE 11: Adverse Reactions of Antiretroviral Agents (cont.)

Miscellaneous Reactions	
GI intolerance	
Agent	All PIs: LPV/r ≈ FPV/r > ATV/r, ATV/cobi, > DRV/r, DRV/cobi, SQV/r NRTIs: ZDV > ddI> other NRTIs EVG/COBI/TDF/FTC
ADR Features	Nausea, vomiting, diarrhea, anorexia. Begins with first dose. Diarrhea: LPV/r, NFV, buffered ddI
Frequency	Common
Monitor	Warn patient
Intervention	Symptomatic - may improve with food (except ddI and IDV without RTV); NFV and LPV/r-associated diarrhea is usually managed with loperamide, calcium; many improve with continuation of treatment. Nausea - prochlorperazine or metoclopramide
Cholelithiasis	
Agent	ATV
ADR features	Abd pain; may cause cholecystitis, choledocholithiasis, pancreatitis, cholangitis
Monitoring	Consider RUQ US with abd pain
Intervention	d/c ATV
Peripheral neuropathy	
Agent	ddI and d4T
ADR Features	Paresthesias and pain of lower extremities after weeks to months d4T also associated with rare cases of ascending neuromuscular weakness
Frequency	10-30% (or more) based on duration and dose
Monitor	Warn patient: Symptoms of decreased LE vibratory sensation and ankle jerk reflexes.
Intervention	D/C implicated agent. Possibly reversible if drug stopped early. Symptomatic treatment - pain meds, foot bridge, etc. Reversible if drug stopped early. Treat pain with gabapentin (most expensive), tricyclics, lamotrigine, oxycarbamazepine, tramadol, topiramate, and/or narcotics, topical lidocaine or capsaicin.
Rash	
Agent	NNRTIs (NVP, EFV, ETR, RPV), PI, (ATV, DRV/r, LPV/r, FPV, TPV/r,) InSTI, (RAL, EVG/c), MVC, and ABC
ADR Features	Maculopapular ± pruritus -- Rare cases SJS, TEN
Frequency	NVP & EFV-15%, FPV-20%, ABC-5%, TPV/r-10-14%, ETR-9%, RPV-3%, DRV-7%
Monitor	Warn patient
Intervention	R/O, NNRTI-associated Stevens-Johnson syndrome or TEN and ABC hypersensitivity. Also R/O rash due to HIV-associated dermatologic complications and drug rashes due to other meds especially TMP-SMX, dapsone etc. Can often 'treat through' maculopapular rashes, but must D/C if progressive.

Miscellaneous Reactions (cont.)	
Myopathy	
Agent	AZT>RAL
ADR features	Increased CPK, muscle weakness and rhabdomyolysis
Monitor	Warn patient
Intervention	D/C AZT or RAL
Insulin resistance	
Agent	PIs (especially IDV) except ATV
ADR Features	FBS > 126 mg/dL ± symptoms of diabetes
Frequency	3-5%; higher frequency with family history of diabetes
Monitor	FBS at baseline, 3 mos, and then q3-6mos
Intervention	Switch to NNRTI- or InSTI-based ART regimen.Diet and exercise, metformin or rosiglitazone (no drug interactions with PIs) if indicated; may need insulin.
Hyperlipidemia	
Agent	Rank order to increase lipids: TPV/r>>LPV/r=FPV/r>IDV/r>SQV/r>EFV>DRV/r; ATV/r >ATV; EFV/c/TDF/FTC; RAL
ADR Features	Increased total and LDL cholesterol and triglycerides; Triglycerides esp. high with TPV/r. RTV, LPV/r = FPV/ Begins within weeks.
Frequency	Variable
Monitor	Fasting lipid profile at baseline, 3-6 mos, and then annually.
Intervention	Based on National Cholesterol Education Program (*Stone N. Circulation 2014; 129 Suppl 2: S1-45*). See Page 31 Preferred statins: pitavastatin, atorvastatin, or rosuvastatin (with dose adjustment for co-administration with ARV if necessary.) Consider ART regimen change to InSTI based regimen (DTG, RAL).

ABLE 11: Adverse Reactions of Antiretroviral Agents *(cont.)*

Miscellaneous Reactions (cont.)	
poatrophy	
gent	d4T > AZT, ddI
DR Features	Thinning of buccal fat in face, extremities (prominent veins) and buttocks
requency	Common with long-term use
Monitor	Self-image is most important
ntervention	Avoid or discontinue d4T or AZT early if possible - changes are either slow to reverse or are irreversible. Injectable agents: poly-L-lactic acid (*Sculptra*)
Mental Status Changes Including Depression	
Agent	EFV > RPV; RAL, DTG
ADR Features	Spectrum includes confusion, impaired concentration, dizziness, abnormal dreams and depression. Possible increased risk of suicide or suicidal ideation Insomnia reported with DTG
Frequency	Up to 50% of EFV recipients; less frequent and severe with RPV
Monitor	Warn patient of mental status changes including abnormal dreams; changes are noted immediately and usually improve with continued use over 2-4 weeks. Caution patient regarding driving, operating heavy machinery and jobs requiring high level neurocognitive function. Symptoms reduced with initial EFV dosing on empty stomach since food increases absorption. Symptoms resolve with alternative regimen and usually resolve or improve with switch to RPV.

TABLE 12: Antiretroviral Agents - "Black Box" Warnings

Agent	Reaction
Abacavir	• Fatal upon rechallenge in patients with hypersensitivity reactions: Do not restart if hypersensitivity reaction cannot be ruled out. (No reported cases with negative HLA B*5701 screening) • Lactic acidosis and steatosis*
Atazanavir**	None
Darunavir**	None
Delavirdine	None
Didanosine	• Fatal and nonfatal pancreatitis: Do not restart • Lactic acidosis with steatosis • Fatal lactic acidosis when combined with stavudine in pregnancy
Dolutegravir	None
Efavirenz	None
Elvitegravir	None
Emtricitabine	• Lactic acidosis with steatosis* • HBV flare (HBsAg) when ARV is stopped. May need to treat HBV. • Safety and efficacy for HBV treatment is not established.
Enfuvirtide	None
Indinavir**	None
Lamivudine	• Lactic acidosis with steatosis* • Patients with HIV infection should receive only dosage and formulations appropriate for treatment of HIV (300mg/d). • HBV flare (HBsAg) when ARV is stopped. May need to treat HBV.
Lopinavir**	None
Maraviroc	• Hepatotoxicity with systemic allergic response (rash, ↑IgE)
Nelfinavir	None
Nevirapine	• Hepatotoxicity including fulminant and cholestatic hepatitis & hepatic necrosis, especially in females with baseline CD4 count > 250 cells/mm^3; monitor intensively in first 18 wks of therapy. • Severe, life-threatening skin reaction including toxic epidermal necrolysis (TEN), Stevens-Johnson syndrome, etc. • Do not restart if there is serious liver injury or serious drug reaction.
Raltegravir	• none
Rilpivirine	• none
Ritonavir	• Potentially serious drug interactions with nonsedating antihistamines, sedative hypnotics, antiarrhythmics, or ergot alkaloids (see Table 16)
Saquinavir**	None
Stavudine	• Lactic acidosis with steatosis • Fatal and non-fatal pancreatitis when used with ddI • Fatal lactic acidosis when combined with ddI in pregnancy

*FDA warning with NRTI class; however, unlikely to occur with ABC, FTC, 3TC, TDF, and TAF
**RTV contraindicated drug combinations applies to boosted PIs (PI/r or PI/cobi)

TABLE 12: Antiretroviral Agents - "Black Box" Warnings (*cont.*)

Agent	Reaction
Tenofovir* alafenamide*/ emtricitabine*	•Lactic acidosis with steatosis •Not approved for HBV infection (but active against HBV) •Potential hepatitis flare when TAF is stopped in patients with chronic hepatitis B. Initiate approved anti-HBV therapy if indicated.
Tenofovir DF*	• Lactic acidosis with steatosis* • Flare of HBV (HBsAg) when antiretroviral is stopped. May need to treat HBV. • Use TDF/FTC for PrEP only after confirming patient is HIV-negative
Tipranavir**	• Clinical reports of hepatitis and hepatic decompensation with death. Increased risk of hepatitis in patients with chronic hepatitis due to HBV or HCV. • Fatal and non-fatal intracranial bleed.
Zidovudine	• Hematologic toxicity: anemia & leukopenia • Prolonged use may cause myopathy • Lactic acidosis and steatosis

*FDA warning with NRTI class; however, unlikely to occur with ABC, FTC, 3TC, TDF, and TAF
**RTV contraindicated drug combinations applies to boosted PIs (PI/r or PI/cobi)

TABLE 13: Cardiovascular Health (Kohli P et al. J Am Heart Assoc 2014; 3:e001098)

Category		Intervention
A	Antiplatelet	ASA 81 mg/d if 10 yr clinical atherosclerotic cardiovascular disease risk > 10%
B	Blood pressure	Goal: <140-150/90
C	Cholesterol	See table 14
C	Cigarettes	Prevention
D	Diet	BMI goal 18.5-24.9 kg/m2; waist <40 (male) and <35 (female)
D	Diabetes	Goal: Hgb A1C <5.7%
E	Exercise	Goal: 3 to 4 forty minutes sessions/week
H	Heart failure	Prevention and/or treatment

TABLE 14: 2013 American College of Cardiology and American Heart Association (ACC/AHA) Guideline on the Treatment of Blood Cholesterol to Reduce Atherosclerotic Cardiovascular Risk in Adults (Stone NJ et al. Circulation 2014; 129: S1-S45

Recommendations for statin therapy to prevent atherosclerotic cardiovascular disease are based on 4 "statin benefit groups" listed below

Patient Group	Intensity of Statin Rx	**Recommended Statin w/ ARVs
Clinical atherosclerotic cardiovascular disease (ASCVD): Hx of angina, MI, coronary revascularization, stroke, TIA, or peripheral arterial disease	Age <75: High-intensity statin; lowers LDL-C by ≥ 50% Age >75: Moderate-intensity statin; lowers LDL-C by 30-50%	DTG, RAL, NRTIs, MVC: atorvastatin 80mg*; rosuvastatin 20 mg PI/r, COBI: Start with atorvastatin 10mg, then titrate to 40mg/d OR rosuvastatin 10mg/d, then titrate to 20mg/d DTG, RAL, NRTIs, MVC, PI/r, COBI: atorvastatin 10mg/d; rosuvastatin 10mg/d; pitavastatin 2-4mg/d
Adult (>21 yrs) with Primary elevations of LDL–C >190 mg/dL	High-intensity statin; lowers LDL-C by ≥ 50%	DTG, RAL, NRTIs, MVC: atorvastatin 80mg*; rosuvastatin 20 mg PI/r, COBI: Start with atorvastatin 10mg, then titrate to 40mg/d OR rosuvastatin 10mg/d, then titrate 20mg/d
DM (age 40 to 75) with LDL–C 70 to189 mg/dL and without clinical ASCVD	Moderate-intensity statin; lowers LDL-C by 30-50%	DTG, RAL, NRTIs, MVC, PI/r, COBI: atorvastatin 10mg/d; rosuvastatin 10mg/d; pitavastatin 2-4mg/d
No clinical ASCVD or DM with LDL–C 70 to 189 mg/dL and estimated 10-year ***ASCVD risk >7.5%	Moderate-to-high intensity statin; LDL-C by 30 to ≥ 50%	DTG, RAL, NRTIs, MVC: atorvastatin 10-80mg/d; rosuvastatin 10-20 mg/d PI/r, COBI: Start with atorvastatin 10mg, then titrate up to 40mg/d OR rosuvastatin 10mg/d, then titrate up to 20mg/d

* Atorvastatin may be decreased to 40mg if pt unable to tolerate 80mg
** Statins dosing added by authors based on ARV drug-drug interactions
*** ASCVD risk calculator (http://tools.cardiosource.org/ASCVD-Risk-Estimator/)

TABLE 15: **Drug Combinations That Should Not Be Used**

	Not Recommended	ART Agent	Alternatives
Alpha adrenergic blocker	Alfuzosin	RTV, DLV*, all PIs*, COBI*	Tamsulosin or doxazosin
Anti-angina	Ranolazine	All PIs*and PI/c, DLV	None
Antiarrhythmic	Flecainide, propafenone	LPV/r, RTV, TPV/r, DRV/r, SQV/r, all PIs*, COBI*	None
	Dofetilide	DTG, all PIs*, COBI*	
	Amiodarone, quinidine, dronedarone	IDV, NFV, RTV, SQV/r, DRV/r, TPV/r, all PIs*, COBI*	
Anti-convulsants	Carbamazapine, oxcarbazepine, phenobarbital, phenytoin	Unboosted PI*, DTG, ETR*, RPV*, EVG/c	Levetiracetam
Anti-gout	Allopurinol	ddI	Alternative NRTI
Antihistamine	Astemizole, terfenadine	All PIs, DLV, EFV, COBI*	Loratadine, cetirizine, fexofenadine, or desloratadine
Antimycobacterial	Rifampin	All PIs and NNRTIs are contraindicated (except EFV) COBI, EVG*, MVC#, TAF	Use rifabutin with PIs§ or Use rifampin with EFV 600 mg qhs, RAL 800mg bid; DTG 50 mg bid
	Rifabutin	DLV, TAF	Clarithromycin, azithromycin
	Rifapentine	All PIs*, NVP*, DLV*, EFV*, ETR*, RPV*, COBI*, EVG*, TAF	Rifabutin (except TAF)
Antineoplastics	Irinotecan	ATV, IDV; caution with other PIs	None
Beta2-Agonist	Salmeterol	RTV, LPV/r, all PI/r*	Formoterol
Ca++ channel blocker	Bepridil	RTV, TPV/r, SQV/r, DRV/r, all PIs*, EFV, COBI*	None
Ergot alkaloid	Ergotamine	All PIs, DLV*, EFV, COBI	Sumatriptan
GI	Cisapride	All PIs, DLV, EFV	Metoclopramide
	Proton pump inhibitor	ATV, NFV, RPV	H2 blocker 12hrs after ATV, NFV, RPV

(continued)

* Added by authors based on pharmacokinetic principles and/or high potential for toxicity
§ See Drug Table 16 (page 36) for rifabutin and antiretroviral dose adjustments
† IV Midazolam may be used with caution as a single dose given for a procedure (w/ LPV/r, ATV/r, TPV/r).
# MVC 600 mg bid can be considered (limited clinical data)

TABLE 15: **Drug Combinations That Should Not Be Used** (*cont.*)

Class	Not Recommended	ART Agent	Alternatives
Hep C drugs	Ribavirin; simeprevir, sofosbuvir, lepidasvir, paritaprevir/rtv dasabuvir ombitasvir, boceprevir	See Table 18 (page 49)	
Herbs	St. John's wort	All PIs, DLV, EFV*, ETR*, NVP*, RPV, COBI, DTG, TAF	Alternative antidepressants
Lipid lowering	Simvastatin, lovastatin	All PIs*, DLV, COBI	Pitavastatin, pravastatin, or dose adjusted atorvastatin, rosuvastatin
Neuroleptic	Pimozide	All PIs, DLV, EFV, COBI	None
Psychotropic	Oral midazolam†, triazolam	All PIs, DLV, EFV	Temazepam, oxazepam or lorazepam
	Alprazolam	DLV, IDV, all PIs*	
	Trazodone	SQV/r, all PIs*, COBI*	
	Lurasidone	all RTV and COBI boosted PIs*, EVG/c	Consider aripiprazole at 25-50% fo the dose with PI/r
Pulmonary HTN Agent	High-dose sildenafil	RTV, LPV/r, all PI/r*, COBI	Dose-adjusted bosentan or tadalafil
Steroid	Dexamethasone (multiple doses)	RPV, All PIs*, NNRTI*, EVG*, COBI*	Prednisone
	Inhaled and intranasal fluticasone	FPV/r, LPV/r, RTV, SQV/r, TPV/r*, ATV*, DRV/r*, all PIs*, COBI*	Beclomethasone

* Added by author based on pharmacokinetic principles and/or high potential for toxicity

TABLE 16: **Drug Interactions: Drug Combinations w/ ARVs**

Class	Agent	ART / Modification
Antifungal	Itraconazole	• All PIs and COBI may increase itra: monitor for toxicities • LPV/r: itraconazole dose > 200 mg/d requires TDM • MVC: 150 mg bid • RPV may be increased,monitor QTc • EFV decreases itraconazole levels; NVP and ETR may decrease itraconazole. TDM recommended
	Ketoconazole	• COBI: COBI and ketoconazole may be increased. IDV/r 800/100 mg bid; ketoconazole ≤ 200 mg/d • MVC: 150 mg bid
		• LPV/r, TPV/r, FPV/r, DRV/r, RTV: ketoconazole ≤ 200 mg/d • FPV: ketoconazole ≤ 400 mg/d
		• NVP: Consider fluconazole as an alternative • RPV AUC ↑ 49%, ketoconazole AUC ↓ 24%, monitor QTc
	Voriconazole	• RTV ≥ 400 mg bid is contraindicated. With boosted PIs (RTV 100-200mg/d), vori AUC decreased by 39%. Voriconazole TDM recommended. • With unboosted PIs, vori and PIs may be increased • EFV 300 mg qhs + voriconazole 400 q12h • COBI may increase vori levels. Voriconazole may increase COBI levels. Voriconazole TDM recommended • Monitor for toxicities. Lower dose RTV may be considered with voriconazole or use alternative. • ETR AUC increase 36% • RPV may be increased, monitor QTc • MVC 150 mg bid
	Fluconazole	• ETR AUC increase 86%; fluconazole – no change • NVP AUC increase 110%; monitor for ADR • PI/r; EFV, RAL, MVC, DTG use standard dose • With TPV/r co-administration do not exceed fluconazole 200 mg/d • RPV may be increased, monitor QTc
	Posaconazole	• ATV and posaconazole levels are increased. Monitor posaconazole concentrations • RPV may be increased, monitor QTc • FPV and posa levels decreased. Avoid • COBI and RTV boosted PIs: Posa may be increased. Recommend TDM • EFV decreased posa AUC 50%. Recommend TDM • ETR and RPV may be increased.
	Anidulafungin Caspofungin Micafungin AmphoB Lipid Ampho Flucytosine Pentamidine	• Limited data. Drug-drug interaction unlikely • No change in caspofungin level with NFV co-administration. • Caspofungin level may be decreased with NVP, EFV, ETR. Consider caspofungin 70mg/d. • Monitor closely for nephrotoxicity with IV pentamidine or amphoB and TDF co-administration.

(continued)

TABLE 16: Drug Interactions: Drug Combinations w/ARVs

(cont.)

Class	Agent	ART / Modification
Opiate	Buprenorphine	• EFV, ETR: small decrease in buprenorphine conc.; no withdrawal symptoms observed. • ATV: increase buprenorphine, decrease ATV. Avoid • ATV/r, DRV/r: increase buprenorphine. Monitor • TPV/r: decrease TPV and buprenorphine active metabolite • NVP (and likely RPV), LPV/r, FPV/r, DTG, RAL: usual dose
	Fentanyl	• PI/r, COBI, DLV: may significantly increase fentanyl concentration. Avoid or use with very close monitoring
	Methadone	• NVP and EFV: significantly decrease methadone by 50%; monitor for withdrawal • ETR: no interaction • RPV: R-methadone decreased 16% • IDV and ATV: no interaction • TPV/r>LPV/r>ATV/r, FPV/r, SQV/r, DRV/r: may decrease methadone levels and require monitoring for withdrawal, but clinical significance is unclear • Methadone decreases buffered ddI levels; use ddI EC (no interaction) • AZT AUC increased 29-43%. Monitor for toxicity • MVC: no interaction • DTG, EVG, RAL, COBI: no significant interaction
	Meperidine	• RTV: nor-meperidine increase 47%. Monitor
	Morphine, Hydromorphone	• RTV (at steady-state) may decrease morphine concentrations. Titrate to effect.
	Oxycodone	• LPV/r: oxycodone increase 2.6-fold. With PI/r, use low dose and monitor for sedation.
Benzodia-zepines	Midazolam Triazolam	• PI/r, COBI, EFV, DLV: Contraindicated with oral midazolam and triazolam. Use lorazepam, oxazepam, or temazepam. • Use single dose IV midazolam w/ caution; consider propofol for procedural sedation.
	Diazepam Clorazepam Chlordiazepoxide Estazolam Flurazepam	• PI/r, COBI, DLV: Benzo may be increased. Consider lorazepam, oxazepam, or temazepam • EFV, NPV, ETR: may decrease benzo. Titrate to effect • DTG, RAL, RPV, MVC, NRTIs: interaction unlikely
	Lorazepam Oxazepam Temazepam	• PI/r, NNRTIs, INSTIs, MVC: interaction unlikely.
Hypnotics	Eszopiclone, Zaleplon, Zolpidem; Suvorexant	• RTV: zolpidem increased 27%. Use low dose zolpidem with PI/r and COBI • PI/r and COBI: no data. Hypnotics may be increased. Consider temazepam or low dose zolpidem. • Suvorexant not recommended with PI and COBI.

(continued)

TABLE 16: Drug Interactions: Drug Combinations w/ARVs (cont.)

Class	Agent	ART / Modification
Anti mycobacterial	Rifabutin**	• All boosted PIs: standard dose PI/r + RBT 150 mg qd or 300 mg 3x/wk (monitor RBT levels) • Note: recommended dose higher than FDA labeling because HIV-infected pts have lower RBT exposures. • Unboosted PI (ATV, FPV, IDV, NFV): RBT 150 mg/d or 300 mg 3x/wk (monitor RBT levels). Consider boosted PIs. • EFV 600 mg/d +RBT 450-600 mg/d or 600 mg 3x/wk • RPV: RBT 300 mg qd plus RPV 50 mg qd • ETR, NVP, RAL, DTG, MVC: RBT 300 mg qd; standard ARV dose • EVG/c: RBT metabolite increased 625%, EVG Cmin decreased 67%. Avoid • ATV/c, DRV/c: RBT 150 mg every other day. Monitor RBT levels
	Rifampin	• All PIs & NNRTIs: contraindicated except EFV (600 mg/d) using standard doses of rifampin • NVP, ETR, RPV: Contraindicated • EVG/c, ATV/c, DRV/c: Contraindicated • MVC: Avoid. Consider MVC 600 mg bid or use rifabutin • RAL: avoid or increase RAL to 800 mg bid • DTG: increase DTG to 50 m bid. Use only in pts with no INSTI mutations.
	Rifapentine	• May significantly decrease PIs, NNRTIs, DTG, RAL, EVG. Avoid
	Bedaquiline	• LPV/r: bedaquiline AUC increased 22%. Monitor QTc • COBI, PIs & DLV: May increase bedaquiline levels. Use only if benefit outweighs risk. Monitor QTc and LFTs
Erectile Dysfunction Agents***	Avanafil	• RTV increased avanafil AUC 13-fold. Avoid all boosted PIs, DLV, and COBI.
	Sildenafil	• COBI, PIs & DLV: ≤ 25 mg q48h and monitor • MVC and RAL: No data; interaction unlikely • ETR: Sildenafil AUC decreased 57%. Titrate
	Vardenafil	• COBI, PIs & DLV: ≤ 2.5 mg q72h
	Tadalafil	• COBI, PIs & DLV: start with 5 mg; do not exceed 10 mg/72h

* Do not co-administer ETR with DRV/r or SQV/r when combined with rifabutin

** For the treatment of TB, most experts recommend rifabutin 150 mg qd with PI/r. Consider rifabutin TDM.

*** Interaction unlikely with RPV, DTG, RAL, MVC. With ETR, NVP, EFV ED agents level may decrease.

(continued)

TABLE 16: Drug Interactions: Drug Combinations w/ARVs (cont.)

Class	Agent	ART / Modification
Lipid lowering agent	Simvastatin Lovastatin	• EFV: simvastatin decrease 68%. With EFV, ETR, NVP: may require simvastatin and lovastatin dose increase. • All boosted PIs and COBI: up to 30-fold increase. Contraindicated. Use pitavastatin, atorvastatin • RPV, DTG, RAL, MVC, all NRTIs: standard dose
	Atorvastatin	• All PIs and COBI may substantially increase atorvastatin levels -- 8-fold with TPV/r (avoid) and LPV/r; 4-fold with DRV/r; 2.5-fold with FPV/r. Start with possible dose of atorvastatin (10 mg). • EFV, ETR, (and NVP): may reduce atorvastatin levels by ~1/3 • RPV: no interaction • RAL, DTG, MVC, all NRTIs: interaction unlikely
	Pitavastatin	• No dose change for most agents. • ATV: pitavastation conc. increase 31% • DRV/r, LPV/r: no clinically significant change.
	Pravastatin	• No dose change for most agents. • EFV, NFV: pravastatin decreased; clinical significance unknown, may need to increase pravastatin dose • DRV/r, pravastatin AUC increases in some patients 81%, but can be up to 5X in others • LPV/r: pravastatin AUC increase 33%; monitor. • MVC: No data; use standard doses • DTG, RAL: interaction unlikely • COBI: no data.
	Rosuvastatin	• Rosuvastatin AUC ↑ 108% (w/ LPV/r), ↑ 213% (w/ ATV/r), ↑ 26% (w/ TPV/r). Dose: 5-10mg/day • DRV/r, FPV, SQV/r: Rosuvastatin AUC ↑ possible -- start 5 mg/d with slow titration. • COBI: Rosuvastatin AUC increase 38%. • DTG, RAL, RPV, MVC: interaction unlikely • FPV: no interaction
	Cholestyramine/ Colesevelam	• Binds to both basic and acidic drugs. No data with ARVs, but ARV absorption may be affected. Avoid co-administration.
	Fenofibrate	• ARV drug-drug interaction unlikely
	Gemfibrozil	• ARV drug-drug interaction unlikely
	Niacin	• ARV drug-drug interaction unlikely
	Omega-3 acid ethyl esters	• ARV drug-drug interaction unlikely
	Ezetimibe	• No interaction with LPV/r. Interaction with other ARVs unlikely.

* Contraindicated with EFV, but clinical significance unknown

(continued)

TABLE 16: **Drug Interactions: Drug Combinations w/ARVs** *(cont.)*

Class	Agent	ART / Modification
Antidepressants	SSRIs (Citalopram, Escitalopram, Fluvoxamine Fluoxetine Paroxetine Sertraline)	• EFV and DRV/r: sertraline decrease 39% and 49%, respectively. Titrate to effect. • DRV/r and FPV/r: Paroxetine decrease 39% and 55%, respectively. EFV and ETR: no interaction. • RTV: no interaction with escitalopram • With NNRTIs and PIs, titrate SSRI to effect.
	SNRIs (Duloxetine, Milnacipran, Venlafaxine, Desvenlafaxine)	• Duloxetine may be increased with PI/r. At steady-state PI/r may decrease duloxetine • Venlafaxine may be increased with PI/r. The active metabolite Desvenlafaxine and milnacipran may be increased with ATV/r, but decreased with PI/r and NFV. • Interaction unlikely with MVC, DTG, RAL
	TCAs (Amitriptyline, Clomipramine Desipramine, Doxepin, Imipramine, Nortriptyline) TetraCAs (Maprotiline Mirtazapine)	• RTV: Avoid desipramine co-administration • RTV or COBI boosted PI may ↑ TCA concentrations. Use with close monitor for ADRs (QTc prolongation, sedation) • SSRIs are preferred over TCAs with PI/r co-administration. • PI/r and COBI: may increase mirtazapine levels. Use low dose and titrate to effect.
	Bupropion	• LPV/r: bupropion ↓ 46%; • EFV: bupropion ↓ 55%
	Trazodone, Nefazodone	• LPV/r: trazodone increased 240%. Wth PI/r start with low dose and monitor for CNS ADR and cardiac arrhythmias. • SQV/r: contraindicated w/ trazodone • PI/r and COBI: nefazodone may be significantly increased. Use with caution (monitor LFTs).
Antipsychotic	Fluphenazine, Haloperidol, Loxapine Perphenazine, Pimozide Thioridazine,	• PI/r, COBI: contraindicated with pimozide • PI/r, COBI: may increase typical antipsychotic levels. Start with low dose and monitor for ADR (QTc prolongation, anticholinergic, EPS) • RPV: with PI/r or COBI administration with typical antipsychotic, monitor for QTc prolongation. • EFV, NVP: may decrease pimozide • DTG, RAL, MVC, NRTIs: Interaction unlikely
	Aripiprazole, Clozapine, Lurasidone, Olanzapine, Paliperidone, Quetiapine, Risperidone, Ziprasidone	• PI/r, COBI: may increase aripiprazole,quetiapine, risperidone, ziprasidone. Monitor QTc with ziprasidone co-administration. • PI/r, COBI: significant (>9-fold) increase in lurasidone; avoid. • PI/r: may decrease clozapine and olanzapine at steady-state. • PI/r, COBI, NNRTIs: Interaction with paliperidone unlikely • EFV, NVP: may decrease lurasidone, quetiapine, aripiprazole, risperidone, ziprasidone. • RPV: monitor QTc with ziprasidone when PI/r is co-administered • DTG, RAL, NRTIs, MVC: interaction unlikely

TABLE 16: **Drug Interactions: Drug Combinations w/ARVs** *(cont.)*

Class	Agent	ART / Modification
Stimulants	Atomoxetine, Dextroamphetamine, Lisdexamfetamine, Methylphenidate, , Modafinil	• PI/r, COBI: may increase modafinil, D-amphetamine, atomoxetine. • Modafinil may decrease PIs, COBI, EVG, MVC, RPV levels • Methylphenidate: not data, interaction unlikely
GI agents	Antacid	• Avoid co-administration with ATV, RPV, NFV, TPV/r. • Give antacid 4 hrs after RPV, ATV, NFV, TPV/r • EVG, RAL, DTG: decreased by ~50-70%. Give EVG or DTG >2hrs before antacid • Avoid Al and Mg antacids with RAL • Although manufacturer recommends CaCO3 w/ RAL, RAL AUC decreased by 54%. Avoid or use with close VL monitoring.
	H-2 Blocker	• ATV: Administer ATV 2h before or 10h after H2 blocker or use ATV/r 300/100 (in PI-naive patients); in treatment-experienced patients, boost with RTV and give H2 blocker (do not exceed equivalent of famotidine 20 mg) separately; consider alternative. ATV/r 400/100 if used with H2 blocker and TDF • RPV: H2 blocker 12 hrs before or 4 hrs after RPV • EVG/c, RAL, DTG: no interaction
	PPI	• Unboosted ATV, NFV, DLV, and RPV: avoid • ATV/r: avoid in PI-experienced pts. In PI-naive, avoid if possible. If needed, do not exceed omeprazole 20 mg equivalent. • RAL AUC increased 212%. Use standard dose • No significant interaction with DTG, EVG/c, LPV/r, FPV/r, EFV, NVP
	Dolasetron Granisatron Ondansetron	• ARV interaction unlikely; use standard dose
	Low dose erythromycin	• EVG, COBI, PIs, NVP may be increased • COBI, PI/r, DLV may increase erythromycin. Monitor QTc • RPV may be increased. Monitor QTc
	Prochlorperazine Metoclopramide Dronabinol	• Significant ARV drug-drug interactions unlikely with dronabinol. • Metoclopramide may be decreased with PI/r at steady-state. • Prochlorperazine: no data; use low dose with PI/r and titrate.

TABLE 16: **Drug Interactions: Drug Combinations w/ARVs** *(cont.)*

Class	Agent	ART / Modification
Diabetes agents	Glipizide Glyburide	• PI/r, DLV, and COBI: glipizide and glyburide may be increased.
	Nateglinide Repaglinide	• PI/r, DLV, and COBI may increase nateglinide and significantly increase repaglinide. A 19-fold increase in repaglinide observed with other CYP3A4 inhibitor (itraconazole). Nateglinide preferred • ETR, EFV, NVP: may decrease repaglinide and nateglinide. Titrate to effect
	Pioglitazone Rosiglitazone	• Pioglitazone may be increased with PI/r, DLV, COBI. • LPV/r, NFV, EFV levels were not significantly affected by rosiglitazone. Rosiglitazone preferred with PI/r.
	Acarbose Miglitol	• ARV drug-drug interactions unlikely
	Sitagliptin Saxagliptin Linagliptin	• PI/r, COBI, NRTI, NNRTI: drug-drug interaction unlikely with sitagliptin • PI/r and COBI: Saxagliptin level may be significantly increased with PI/r, COBI, do not exceed 2.5 mg/day • Linagliptin: PI/r and COBI may moderately increase linagliptin level
	Metformin	• DTG: may increase metformin concentrations. Use with caution or avoid with renal insufficiency.
Antihistamine	Astemizole Terfenadine (off the market)	• Contraindicated with PI/r, DLV, and COBI. • Cetirizine, desloratidine, fexofenadine, loratidine can be used with PI/r and COBI.
Antigout	Allopurinol	• Avoid ddI. • No ARV drug-drug interaction with other NRTIs
	Colchicine	• Avoid colchicine with PI/r and COBI with renal and hepatic impairment. • With co-administration: Administer colchicine 0.6 x 1, then 0.3 mg one hour later for gout flare. Co-administer only when PI/r is at steady-state (10-14 days).

TABLE 16: **Drug Interactions: Drug Combinations w/ARVs** *(cont.)*

Class	Agent	ART / Modification
Anti-convulsant	Phenobarbital, Phenytoin, Carbamazepine Oxcarbazepine	• Combinations of boosted PIs with designated anticonvulsants should be avoided or given with caution and monitoring of anticonvulsant and PI levels or consider valproic acid or levetiracetam† • Avoid unboosted PIs, once-daily LPV/r, and NNRTI • RPV is contraindicated • Carbamazepine: ↓ IDV and potentially other PIs (except DRV) and NNRTIs • Phenytoin: ↓ NFV, ↓ LPV, and potentially other PIs (except FPV/r) and NNRTIs. Phenytoin levels also ↓ with NFV, FPV/r, and LPV/r. Monitor level. • MVC: 600 mg bid • RAL: close monitoring with phenytoin and phenobarbital • EVG and DTG may be decreased • TAF may be decreased. Avoid
	Valproic acid	• LPV AUC ↑ 38%, TPV/r may ↓ valproic acid • EFV: no change
	Lamotrigine	• LPV/r: lamotrigine AUC decrease 50% • ATV/r: lamotrigine AUC decreased 32%; unboosted ATV: no change
	Ethosuximide	• PI/r, DLV, COBI may increase ethosuximide level • NVP, EFV, ETR may decrease ethosuximide level
	Zonisamide	• PI/r, DLV, COBI may increase zonisamide level • NVP, EFV, ETR may decrease zonisamide level
	Levitiracetam Topiramate	• ARV drug-drug interaction unlikely
Antibiotic	Clarithromycin	• DLV, DRV/r, LPV/r, RTV, SQV/r, TPV/r, COBI: decrease clarithromycin dose in renal failure or use azithromycin. • ATV increases clari level; decrease clari dose by 50% • MVC: 150 mg bid • ETR, EFV, NVP: may decrease clari levels; May increase RPV; consider azithromycin • DTG, EVG may be increased. • RAL: interaction unlikely • Consider using azithromycin (no interaction)
	ABX that are Non-CYP3A4 substrates or inhibitors, or inducer	• Interaction with ARVs unlikely with the following abx: aminoglycosides, beta-lactams, carbapenems, cephalosporins, clindamycin, ethambutol, fluoroquinolones, sulfadiazine, sulfamethoxazole, vancomycin • Isoniazid, linezolid, metronidazole: monitor for neuropathy with long-term co-administration with ddI or d4T.

TABLE 16: Drug Interactions: Drug Combinations w/ARVs *(cont.)*

Class	Agent	ART / Modification
Anti-parasitics	Artemether/ Lumefantrine	• DRV/r, LPV/r: ~18% decrease in artemeter and 2-3-fold increase in lumefantrine concentrations. Monitor for ARV efficacy and ADR. • PI/c and EVG/c : may increase lumefantrine levels. • EFV: artemether active metabolite decrease 75% and lumefantrine decrease 56%. Monitor closely for efficacy. • ETR: artemether active metabolite decrease 15% nd lumefantrine decrease 13%. • NVP: artemether active metabolite decrease 37%. Lumafantrine AUC decreased 25% in one study and increased 55.6% in another. Monitor closely for efficacy.
Anti-parasitics	Atovaquone/ proguanil	• EFV, LPV/r, ATV/r lower atovaquone AUC by 75%, 74%, 46% respectively. • Proguanil concentrations decrease by 38-43%. • Consider alternative malaria prophylaxis
Anti-parasitics	Mefloquine	• RTV AUC decrease 31%. Monitor for boosted PI antiviral efficacy.
Anti-parasitics	Quinine	• RTV: quinine concentrations increased 4-fold • LPV/r: quinine AUC decrease by 50%. • PI/r, COBI: Monitor for therapeutic efficacy and toxicity (QTc prolongation and cinchonism)
Anti-parasitics	Tinidazole	• PI/r and COBI: may increase tinidazole level. Clinical significance unknown; use standard dose
Anti-parasitics	Albendazole, amodiaquine, dapsone, paromomycin, pyrimethamine	• ARV interaction unlikely; use standard dose
BPH agents	Alpha blocker: alfuzosin, terazosin, doxazosin, tamsulosin	• PI/r, COBI: alfuzosin contraindicated; doxazosin-avoid; terazosin-no data. • PI/r, COBI: tamsulosin may be increased. Start with low dose and warn patient of orthostatic hypotension. • DTG, RAL, NRTIs, MVC, RPV: interaction unlikely • NVP, EFV: may decrease alfuzosin, doxazosin, and tamsulosin level. Titrate to effect.
BPH agents	5-alpha reductase inhibitor: Finasteride Dutasteride	• PI/r, COBI: finasteride and dutasteride levels may be increased. • NVP, EFV: finasteride and dutasteride levels may be decreased. • DTG, RAL, NRTIs, MVC, RPV: interaction unlikely

TABLE 16: Drug Interactions: Drug Combinations w/ARVs (cont.)

Class	Agent	ART / Modification
Anti-neoplastics	Antimetabolite (capecitabine, floxuridine, methotrexate)	• AZT: additive bone marrow suppression • PI/r, NNRTI, COBI, InSTI, MVC: interaction unlikely. Use standard dose.
	Cisplatin, oxaliplatin, hydroxyurea, mitomycin	• Hydroxyurea: increased toxicity (pancreatitis, neuropathy, lactic acidosis) with ddI co-administration. • AZT: additive bone marrow suppression • PI/r, NNRTI, COBI, InSTI, MVC: interaction unlikely. Use standard dose.
	Camptothecin (irinotecan and topotecan)	• IDV, ATV: avoid co-administration with irinotecan • Interaction with topotecan unlikely
	Alkylating agent (Busulfan, cyclophosphamide, dacarbazine, ifosfamide, lomustine, thiotepa) Anthracycline (daunorubicin, doxorubicin, idarubicin)	• IDV: cyclophosphamide clearance decreased by 50%. No change in IDV level. • PI/r, DLV, COBI: may increase alkylating agents levels. • EFV, NVP, ETR: may decrease alkylating agents levels • MVC, RAL, DTG: interaction unlikely • Good clinical outcome observed with standard dose CHOP+PI-based regimen. Modified CHOP (50% of cyclophosphamide and doxorubicin) also effective, but higher rate of relapse.
	Antiandrogen (bicalutamide, flutamide, nilutamide) Aromastase inhibitor (anastozole, exemestane, letrozole) Bexarotene Estrogen receptor antagonist (fulvestrant) Ixabepilone Mitoxantrone Podophyllotoxin (Etoposide, Teniposide) Estrogen Modulator (tamoxifen, toremifene) Tyrosine Kinase Inhibitor (dasatinib, erlotinib, gefitinib, imatinib, lapatinib, sunitinib)	• PI/r, DLV, COBI: may increase chemo agents levels. • EFV, NVP, ETR: may decrease chemo agents levels • RPV, MVC, RAL, DTG: interaction unlikely

Class	Agent	ART / Modification
Antineoplastics (cont)	Taxane (docetaxel, paclitaxel) Temsirolimus	• PI/r, DLV, COBI: may significantly increase taxane levels. Severe toxicity reported with LPV/r and DLV co-administration with paclitaxel. Significant (2-3 fold) increase in temsirolimus expected. • EFV, NVP, ETR: may decrease taxane levels • MVC, RAL, DTG, RPV: interaction unlikely
	Vinca Alkaloid (vinblastine, vincristine, vinorelbine)	• ddI, d4T: may increase the risk of peripheral neuropathy with long-term co-administration. • PI/r, DLV, COBI: may increase vinca alkaloid levels. • EFV, NVP, ETR: may decrease vinca alkaloid levels • MVC, RAL, DTG, RPV: interaction unlikely
Anti-Arrhythmic	Disopyramide IV lidocaine Mexilitine Procainamide	• PI/r, COBI, DLV: may increase anti-arrhythmic levels. Use with caution and monitor closely • ETR, EFV, NVP: may decrease anti-arrhythmic levels. • RAL, DTG, MVC, NRTIs: interaction unlikely • RPV: monitor QTc closely
	Flecainide Propafenone Dofetilide Amiodarone, Quinidine Dronedarone	• PI/r, COBI, DLV: avoid co-administration. • ETR, EFV, NVP: may decrease anti-arrhythmic levels. • RAL, DTG, MVC, NRTIs: interaction unlikely • RPV: monitor QTc closely
Oral Contraceptive	Ethinyl Estradiol Norgestimate Levonorgestrel	• DRV/r, EFV, FPV +/-RTV, LPV/r, NFV, NVP, SQV/r, TPV/r, and RTV: additional method of contraception recommended • ATV/r: use at least 35 mg EE • IDV & ATV: do not exceed 30 mg EE • RPV, DTG, ETR, MVC, and RAL: no interaction • EVG/c may increase norgestimate and decreases EE • ATV/c and DRV/c: no data. • EFV decreases levonorgestrel (PlanB) 58%
	Etonogestrel (releasing subdermal implant)	• LPV/r: etonogestrel AUC increased 52%. Use standard dose. No data with other ARVs. • EFV: etonogestrel AUC decreased 63%. Use additional form of contraception.
	Ethinyl estradiol/ norelgestromin (transdermal)	• LPV/r: no change in LPV. ethinyl estradiol AUC ↓ 45%, norelgestromin AUC ↑ 83%. Use standard dose.

TABLE 16: **Drug Interactions: Drug Combinations w/ARVs** *(cont.)*

Class	Agent	ART / Modification
Ca++ channel blockers	Bepridil	• Contraindicated with all boosted PIs, COBI, and DLV, EFV*
	Diltiazem Amlodipine and other Ca channel blockers	• ATV/r: diltiazem AUC increase 125% • IDV: amlopidine AUC increase 89.8% • With PI/r and COBI: start low dose Ca channel blocker and titrate. Decrease diltiazem dose by 50% and monitor EKG • EFV decrease diltiazem AUC 69%; titrate to effect with EFV, NVP, ETR.
Beta-blockers	Metoprolol Timolol Carvedilol Labetolol Propranolol	• LPV/r, ATV/r: may prolong PR interval. Use with ECG monitoring in pts with known conduction abnormalities. • All PI/r and COBI: may increase beta-blocker concentration
	Atenolol Nadolol Bisoprolol	• LPV/r, ATV/r: may prolong PR interval. Use with ECG monitoring in pts with known conduction abnormalities. • COBI: Pharmacokinetic interaction unlikely.
	Sotalol	• PI/r and COBI: Pharmacokinetic interaction unlikely. • RPV: may prolong QTc. Use with close monitoring
ACE inhibitors	Captopril, Enalapril, Benazepril, Ramipril, Lisinopril	• PI/r, DLV, COBI: may increase captopril, enalapril, benazepril, ramipril. Use low dose and titrate to effect. Interaction unlikely with lisinopril.
ARBs	Losartan, Valsartan, Candesartan, Irbesartan.	• PI/r, DLV, COBI: may increase losartan. Consider candesartan, irbesartan.
Misc Cardiovascular	Clonidine, Hydralazine	• ARV Interaction unlikely with clonidine and hydralazine
	Ranolazine	• PI/r, DLV, COBI: contraindicated • NVP, ETR, EFV: may decrease ranolazine level
	Nitrates	• PI/r, DLV, COBI: may increase isosorbide mononitrate/dinitrate
	Digoxin	• SQV/r and DRV/r: increases digoxin 49% and 36%, respectively. Other PI/r may increase digoxin level. Monitor • COBI: no significant change in AUC. Use standard dose

* Contraindicated with EFV, but clinical significance unknown

TABLE 16: Drug Interactions: Drug Combinations w/ARVs (cont.)

Class	Agent	ART / Modification
Pulmonary hypertension	Bosentan	• PI/r: significant increase bosertan levels; co-administer bosentan 62.5 mg only after PI/r has been given for at least 10 days. • COBI: same bosentan dosing recommendations as with PI/r coadministration, but no data. Co-administer with caution. • NVP, ETR, ERV: may decrease bosentan levels • RPV, MVC, DTG, RAL, all NRTIs: Interaction unlikely
	Tadalafil Sildenafil	• PI/r and COBI: avoid high dose sildenafil • PI/r and COBI: after >7 days on PI/r or COBI, tadalafil 20mg/d (max 40mg/day). No data with COBI; co-administer with caution. • NVP, ETR, EFV: may decrease tadalafil and sildenafil. titrate to effect. • RPV, RAL, DTG, MVC: interaction unlikely. Use standard dose
Glucocorticoid	Systemic steroid	• RTV: prednisone active metabolite increased 31%. • PI/r and COBI: may increase methylprednisolone, triamcinolone, prednisolone. Dose adjustment may be required with long term co-administration. • PIs, RPV, NNRTIs, EVG, DTG, COBI may be decreased by dexamethasone at steady-state. Use alternative corticosteroid with >10 days co-administration.
	Inhaled/ Intranasal steroid	• PI/r and COBI: significant increase in fluticasone serum concentrations resulting in Cushing's and adrenal insufficiency. Avoid • Budesonide levels may be increased. Avoid • Intranasal mometasone: no data; low systemic exposure • Beclomethasone preferred.
Migraine Agents	Dihydroergotamine Ergoloid mesylates Ergotamine	• All PIs, COBI, EFV, DLV: Contraindicated • NPV, ETR: may decrease ergotamine concentrations • MVC, NRTIs, RPV, RAL, DTG: interaction unlikely
	Almotriptan Elitriptan Naratriptan	• All PIs, COBI, DLV: may significantly increase almotriptan, elitriptan, naratriptan levels. Consider rizatriptan, sumatriptan, zolmitriptan • NVP, ETR, EFV: may decrease almotriptan, elitriptan, naratriptan levels. • MVC, NRTIs, RPV, RAL, DTG: interaction unlikely
	Rizatriptan, Sumatriptan, Zolmitriptan	• Interaction unlikely with ARVs

TABLE 16: **Drug Interactions: Drug Combinations w/ARVs** *(cont.)*

Class	Agent	ART / Modification
Immuno-suppressants	Cyclosporine	• PI/r, COBI, DLV: may significantly increase cyclosporine levels** • Target trough 150-450 ng/mL. Higher rejection rate post-renal transplant. Consider using tacrolimus or sirolimus instead. • EFV, NPV, ETR: may decrease cyclosporine levels
	Everolimus	• PI/r, COBI, DLV: may significantly increase cyclosporine levels**
	Tacrolimus	• PI/r, COBI, DLV: may significantly increase tacrolimus levels** • EFV, NPV, ETR: may decrease tacrolimus levels • Target trough: 5-15 ng/mL (lower rates of rejection with target close to 15mcg/mL)
	Sirolimus	• PI/r, COBI, DLV: may significantly increase sirolimus levels** • EFV, NPV, ETR: may decrease sirolimus levels • Preferred in patients with calcineurin-associated toxicity. • Target trough: 3-12 ng/mL.
	Thalidomide	• Avoid long-term co-administration with ddI and d4T due to potential risk of irreversible peripheral neuropathy.
	Mycophenolate	• NFV AUC decreased 32%. Avoid • ATV, IDV: may increase mycophenolic acid • LPV/r, TPV/r: may decrease mycophenolic acid. • NVP clearance increased. Consider alternative NNRTI • Interaction unlikely with DTG, RAL, NRTI
Anticoagulant	Clopidogrel	• ETR: may decrease the efficacy of clopidogrel; avoid
	Warfarin	• Monitor INR closely if given with any PI or NNRTI (especially EFV or RTV) • PI/r and RTV may decrease INR at steady state • ETR may increase INR • RAL, DTG: interaction unlikely • COBI may increase or decrease INR. Monitor closely
	Dabigatran	• PI/r and COBI: avoid if CrCL <30ml/min. • With co-administration, consider dose separation (2 hours before RTV). Reduce dose to 75 mg bid when CrCL 30-50ml/min
	Rivaroxaban	• All PIs, COBI, and DLV may significantly increase rivaroxaban levels. Avoid • EFV, NVP, ETR: may decrease rivaroxaban levels.
	Apixiban	• PIs, COBI, DLV: no data. May increase apixiban; avoid if possible. If co-administered, use 50% of dose, but avoid if >80 y.o, Scr >1.5, <60kg.
	Ticagrelor Vorapaxar	• PIs, COBI, DLV: no data. May increase ticagrelor and vorapaxar; avoid
	Heparin/ Enoxaparin	• Interaction unlikely. Use standard dose

* ** TPV/r may increase cyclosporine, tacrolimus, sirolimus initially, but at steady-state levels may be decreased

TABLE 17: **Drug Interactions: HCV Antivirals w/ ARVs** (*cont.*)

	PI/r	NNRTIs	InSTI	NRTIs	MVC
Sofosbuvir	DRV/r: SD TPV/r: may decrease SOF; avoid	EFV: SD RPV: SD	RAL: SD	TDF*/FTC: SD	No data; SD likely
Ledipasvir	ATV/r, DRV/r, LPV/r: SD	EFV: Ledipasvir decreased 34%.SD RPV: SD ETR, NVP: Ledipasvir may be decreased	EVG/c: avoid when combined with TDF.	TDF*: SD; monitor for nephrotoxicity when combined with PI/r or EFV.	No data: usual dose likely.
Simepravir	DRV: avoid; increased SIM	EFV: avoid ETR, NVP: no data; avoid RPV: SD	RAL: SD DTG: SD likely	TDF*:SD	No interaction: SD
Dasabuvir, ombitasvir, paritaprevir, ritonavir	DRV/r and LPV/r: Avoid ATV: 300mg/d (without RTV)	EFV: Contraindicated RPV: avoid NVP, ETR: no data; avoid	No data. RAL and DTG SD	Usual dose likely	MVC no data; consider 150 mg bid
Daclastavir	Decrease daclatasvir to 30 mg/day with ATV/r, IDV, NFV Daclatasvir 60mg/d with ATV, FPV, DRV/r	EFV, ETR, and (possibly NVP): increase daclastavir dose to 90mg/d RPV: daclatasvir 60mg/d	DTG, RAL: daclastavir 60 mg/d EVG/c or EVG/r: decrease daclastavir dose to 30mg/d	Daclastavir 60mg/d	Daclastavir 60mg/d; MVC standard dose
Grazoprevir/ Elbasvir	ATV, DRV, LPV/r, SQV, TPV/r: increase grazoprevir/ elbasvir concentrations 2 to 8-fold and may increase risk of LFTs elevation. Avoid PI/r and COBI boosted regimens.	RPV: SD EFV: significant decrease in grazoprevir and elbasvir concentrations. Avoid EFV, ETR and likely NVP.	RAL: SD DTG: grazoprevir AUC decreased 36%; elbasvir not affected.	ABC, FTC, 3TC, TDF, likely TAF: SD	No data: standard dose likely.
Ribavirin	SD	SD	SD	ddI: contraindicated AZT: additive anemia	SD

SD standard dose. *TAF may be considered, but no data.

TABLE 18: **HCV Antivirals Drug Interactions**

	Sofos buvir	Ledipasvir	Simepravir	Dasabuvir Ombitasvir, Paritaprevir, RTV	Daclatasvir
Acid reducing agents	SD	May decrease ledipasvir. Separate antacid by 4h; do not exceed famotidine 40mg bid or omeprazole 20mg/d	SD	SD	SD
CYP3A substrate w/ narrow therapeutic index (see page 32-33)	SD	SD	May increase intestinal CYP3A4 substrates (oral midazolam)	Same contraindication with drugs listed for RTV. See page 32-33.	SD
CYP3A4 inhibitors (azole antifungal, macrolides)	SD	SD	May significantly increase simepravir levels. Avoid	Paritaprevir, dasabuvir may be increased. Dose not established.	Decrease daclatasvir to 30 mg/day
Pgp and CYP3A4 inducers (rifampin, St John's wort)	Avoid	Avoid	Avoid	Avoid	Avoid
Anti-convulsants **	Avoid	Avoid	Avoid	Avoid	Avoid
Ethinyl estradiol	No intera ction; SD	No interaction; SD	No interaction; SD	Contraindicated. Potential increased risk of ALT elevation.	SD
Amiodarone	Avoid *	Bradycardia, Avoid	Bradycardia; Avoid	May increase amiodarone levels. Use with close monitoring	Bradycardia; Avoid

SD standard dose;

*bradycardia reported when sofosbuvir (in combination with ledipasvir, simepravir, or daclastavir) was given with amiodarone.

**carbamazepine, phenytoin, phenobarbital, oxcarbazepine

TABLE 19: **Drug Interactions: NRTIs**

Drug	AZT	d4T	ddI	TDF/TAF
Allopurinol	No known interaction	No known interaction	• ddI ↑113 to 312%. Avoid	No known interaction
Atovaquone	AZT AUC ↑31%. Monitor for BM suppression	No known interaction	No known interaction	No known interaction
Cidofovir, ganciclovir, valganciclovir	Ganciclovir + AZT increases marrow toxicity; monitor CBC	No interaction between d4T and ganciclovir	ddI and oral ganciclovir: ddI AUC↑111% (po) and 50-70% (IV); use with caution or avoid	TAF and TDF maybe ↑ May increase levels of co-administered tubular secretion subtrate drugs • Monitor for toxicity
Methadone	AZT AUC ↑43%; no dose change; monitor CBC	d4T ↓27%; no dose change	ddI EC: no interaction	TDF: No change TAF: No data. Interaction unlikely
Ribavirin	Monitor for severe anemia; *in vitro* inhibition of AZT activation; not shown *in vivo*	*In vitro* antagonism but not clinically significant	Magnifies ddI toxicity; contraindicated	• Ribavirin unchanged; no data on TDF level TAF: no data
ddI	Limited clinical data	Increased toxicity: pancreatitis, peripheral neuropathy, lactic acidosis; avoid	--	ddI ↑44% • > 60 kg: 250 mg/d ddI EC • < 60 kg: 200 mg/d ddI EC • Avoid if possible TAF: no data, avoid
ATV	AZT AUC unchanged but C_{min} ↓29%; significance unknown	No interaction based on clinical data	Buffered ddI: take ATV w/ food 2h before or 1h after ddI or use ddI EC; separate dosing due to food restrictions	TDF: • ATV AUC ↓25% • TDF AUC ↑24% • Avoid concomitant use unless ATV/r TAF: TAF AUC ↑91%; ATV <-> Use standard dose
LPV/r	No PK data, but interaction unlikely	No data; interaction unlikely	Take ddI on empty stomach and LPV/r with food	TDF: • TDF AUC ↑32% • Use standard doses and monitor for TDF toxicity TAF: TAF AUC↑47%; LPV <-> Use standard dose
TPV/r	AZT ↓35%; clinical significance unknown	No interaction	Separate dose of ddI EC by ≥ 2h	TDF: • TPV AUC ↓ 9-18% TAF: may ↓ TAF. Avoid.
DRV/r	Interaction unlikely	Interaction unlikely	Take DRV 2h before ddI	TDF: • TDF AUC ↑22% • DRV no change TAF: no change standard dose

TABLE 20: **Dose Adjustments with PIs and NNRTIs Co-Administration**

	EFV	NVP	ETR	RPV§
ATV/r	ATV/r 400/100 (with food) + EFV SD (avoid in PI-experienced pts)	Avoid NVP increase, ATV decrease	ATV ↓14%. Avoid, but unclear clinical significance	RPV 25 qd ATV/r 300/100 qd
ATV/c	ATV/c 400/150 (with food) + EFV SD (avoid in PI-experienced pts)	Avoid NVP may increase, ATV may decrease	Avoid ETR may increase, ATV may decrease	RPV 25 qd ATV/c 300/150 qd
DRV/r	DRV/r 600/100 bid EFV 600 qhs (with DRV mutations); consider TDM	• DRV/r 600/100 bid + NVP 200 bid • NVP ↑27%	DRV/r 600/100 bid + ETR 200 bid	RPV AUC ↑130% DRV SD DRV/r 800/100 po qd + RPV 25 qd
DRV/c	Avoid DRV and COBI may decrease	Avoid NVP may increase, DRV and COBI may decrease	Avoid ETR may increase, DRV and COBI may decrease	RPV 25 qd DRV/c 800/150 qd
FPV	• FPV/r 1400/300 qd + EFV SD • FPV/r 700 bid + RTV 100 bid + EFV 600 qhs	FPV/r 700/100 bid + NVP 200 bid NVP Cmin ↑22%	APV ↑ 69%. Beneficial interaction. Avoid, but unclear clinical significance	FPV/r 700/100 bid or FPV 1400/200 qd + RPV 25 qd
IDV	• IDV 1000 q8h** + EFV 600 qhs; or • IDV 800 q12h + RTV 200 bid + EFV 600 qhs	• IDV 800 q12h + RTV 200 bid + NVP 200 bid	Avoid	IDV/r 800/100 bid + RPV 25 qd
LPV/r	LPV/r 500/125† bid + EFV 600 mg qhs	LPV/r 500/125 bid + NVP SD	LPV/r 400/100 bid + ETR 200 bid	RPV AUC ↑52%, LPV 400/100 bid + RPV 25 qd
NFV	NFV SD + EFV SD	NFV SD + NVP SD ‡	Avoid	SD
SQV	SQV/r 1000/100 bid + EFV 600 mg qhs	SQV/r 1000/100 bid +	SQV/r 1000/100 mg bid + ETR SD	SD
TPV/r	TPV/r 500/200 bid + EFV 600 mg qhs	NVP no change SD	ETR ↓76%; Avoid	SD

* All doses in mg
SD = Standard dose
TDM = Therapeutic drug monitoring
** Suboptimal PK. Boosting with RTV preferred
† LPV/r 600/150 mg bid preferred in treatment-experienced patients
‡ Limited clinical data, dose not established
§ RPV concentrations may be increased with PI/r or PI/cobi. Consider monitoring QTc in patients at risk for QTc prolongation

TABLE 21: **Dose Adjustments with InSTI and NNRTIs or PI Co-Administration**

	DTG	EVG/COBI/ TDF/FTC	EVG/rtv	RAL
ATV/r ATV/c	DTG AUC↑62% w/ ATV/r DTG 50 qd+ ATV/r 300/100 OR ATV 400 qd ATV/c: no data; use SD	No data; avoid	EVG Cmin ↑ 38% w/ ATV/r; EVG 85 +ATV/r 300/100 qd No data w/ ATV/; avoid	RAL AUC ↑41% w/ ATV/r; use SD No data w/ ATV/c; SD likely
DRV/r DRV/c	DTG AUC ↓ 22% w/ DRV/r DTG 50 qd + DRV/r SD DRV/c: no data; use SD	No data; avoid	EVG 150 qd + DRV/r 600/100 bid	RAL 400 bid + DRV/r SD or DRV/c 800/150 qd
FPV+/- RTV	DTG Cmin ↓49% DTG 50 BID + FPV/r SD (use only if no InSTI resistance)	No data; avoid	No interaction EVG 150 qd + FPV/r 700/100 bid	APV: no change RAL 400 bid+ FPV 700/100 bid
IDV	DTG may increase No data; SD	No data; avoid	No data; avoid	RAL may increase No data; SD
LPV/r	DTG: no change DTG 50 qd + LPV/r SD	No data; avoid	EVG AUC ↑ 75% EVG 85 qd + LPV/r 400/100 bid	RAL 400 bid LPV/r 400/100 bid
NFV	No data; SD likely	No data; avoid	No data; avoid	No data; SD likely
SQV/r	No data; SD likely	No data; avoid	No data; dose not established	No data; SD likely
TPV/r	DTG Cmin ↓ 76% DTG 50 BID + TPV/r SD (use only if no INSTI resistance)	No data; avoid	EVG 150 qd + TPV/r 500/200 bid	RAL AUC ↓ 24% RAL 400 bid+ TPV/r 500/200 bid
EFV	DTG AUC ↓57% DTG 50 bid + EFV 600 qhs (use only if no INSTI resistance)	EVG may decrease Avoid	No data. Avoid	RAL AUC ↓ 36% EFV 600 qhs+ RAL 400 bid
ETR	With co-administration, must be given with boosted PI (DRV/r) DTG 50 qd + ETR 200 bid w/ PI/r.	EVG may decrease Avoid	ETR 200 bid + EVG/ATV/r 85/300/100 qd EVG/LPV/r 85/400/100bid EVG/DRV/r 150/600/100 bid	ETR and RAL Cmin ↓ 17% and 34%, respectively. ETR 200 bid + RAL 400 bid
NVP	May ↓ DTG Avoid	May ↓ EVG Avoid	May ↓ EVG Avoid	No data. Usual dose likely
RPV	DTG 50 qd RPV 25 qd	RPV may increase; avoid	RPV may increase SD; monitor QTc	No data. Usual dose likely

SD: standard dose
All drug doses are in mg

TABLE 22: Pharmacokinetic Enhancement Co-administration PI or InSTI with COBI or RTV

	COBI	RTV
ATV	ATV/c 300/150 mg qd (co-formulation)	ATV/r 300/100 mg qd ATV/r 400/100 mg qd (with EFV)
DRV	DRV/c 800/150 mg qd (co-formulation)	DRV/r 800/100 qd DRV/r 600/100 bid
FPV	No data	FPV/r 700/100 bid or FPV/r 1400/100 qd
IDV	No data	IDV/r 800/100 bid
LPV	No data	LPV/r 400/100 mg bid LPV/r 800/200 mg qd (co-formulation)
SQV	No data	SQV/r 1000/100 bid or SQV/RTV 400/400 mg bid
DTG	No data. Minimal DTG boosting expected	Minimal DTG boosting expected
EVG	EVG/COBI/TDF/FTC 150/150/300/200 (co-formulation)	EVG 85 mg qd+ATV/r300/100 mg qd EVG 85 mg qd+LPV/r 400/100 mg bid EVG 150 mg qd+DRV/r/600/100 mg bid EVG 150 mg qd+FPV/r700/100 mg bid EVG 150 mg qd+TPV/r500/200 mg bid
RAL	No boosting effect Use SD w/ COBI	No boosting effect Use SD w/ RTV

SD: standard dose

TABLE 23: Dose Adjustments with InSTI and NNRTIs or PI Co-Administration

Maraviroc dosing when given in combination with PI, COBI, NRTIs, NNRTIs, InSTIs.

	EFV	NVP	ETR	RPV
DTG RAL	MVC 600 mg bid	MVC 300 mg bid	MVC 600 mg bid	MVC 300 mg bid
NRTIs (TDF, ABC, 3TC, FTC)	MVC 600 mg bid	MVC 300 mg bid	MVC 600 mg bid	MVC 300 mg bid
PI/r* (except TPV/r) +/- NRTI	MVC 150 mg bid	MVC 150 mg bid	MVC 150 mg bid	MVC 150 mg bid
TPV/r	MVC 600 mg bid	MVC 300 mg bid	MVC 600 mg bid	MVC 300 mg bid
COBI* +/- NRTI	MVC 150 mg bid	MVC 150 mg bid	MVC 150 mg bid	MVC 150 mg bid
CYP3A4 inhibitor* (e.g Telithromycin, Clarithromycin, Erythromycin, Itraconazole, Ketoconazole, Voriconazole, Delavirdine)	MVC 150 mg bid	MVC 150 mg bid	MVC 150 mg bid	MVC 150 mg bid
CYP3A4 strong inducer (e.g Carbamazepine Phenytoin Phenobarbital)	MVC 600 mg bid	MVC 600 mg bid	MVC 600 mg bid	MVC 600 mg bid
Rifampin Rifapentine	Avoid or consider MVC 600 mg bid	Avoid	Avoid	Avoid
Rifabutin	MVC 600 mg bid	MVC 300 mg bid	MVC 600 mg bid	MVC 300 mg bid

* manufacturer recommends avoiding boosted PI with MVC with CrCL <30ml/min. Although NNRTIs are also not recommended with MVC in patients with CrCL <30ml/in, the clinical significance is unclear.

ANTIRETROVIRAL THERAPY

TABLE 24A: **Indications for ART: DHHS** (Jan. 28, 2016)

ART is recommended for ALL HIV-infected persons to treat HIV infection and to prevent HIV transmission
Strength of recommendation based on rating described in table 24B: CD4 count <350/uL: AI; 350-500/uL: AI; CD4 > 500/uL: AI AIDS-defining conditions, including HAD (HIV-associated dementia) AI Acute opportunistic Infections*: AI Pregnancy: AI Chronic HBV co-infection: AII HIV-associated nephropathy: AII Rapidly declining CD4 count (eg >100 cell/mm³ per year) AIII Acute HIV: BII HCV-coinfection BII Higher viral load (>100,000 c/mL) BII

* Initiate ARVs within 2 weeks of new OI including lymphomas and HPV-associated cancer
An exception is cryptococcal meningitis in which delay initiation of ART until after 10 weeks of induction/consolidation antifungal to avoid the consequences of IRIS. Earlier ARTs start may be considered in pts with severe immunosuppression (CD4 <50)
In TB treatment-naive patients, ART should be started within 2 weeks if baseline CD4 <50/uL and may be delayed to 8-12 weeks if higher (2015 DHHS OI Guidelines).

TABLE 24B: **Rating Scheme for Recommendation**

Strength of Recommendation	Quality of Evidence for Recommendation
A: Strong recommendation for the statement	**I**: One or more randomized trials with clinical outcomes and/or validated laboratory endpoints
B: Moderate recommendation for the statement	**II**: One or more well-designed, non-randomized trials or observational cohort studies with long-term clinical outcomes
C: Optional recommendation for the statement	**III**: Expert opinion

TABLE 25: **What to start: DHHS Guidelines** (Jan. 28, 2016)

Preferred *	Caution
<u>InSTI-based regimens</u> DTG/ABC/3TC (AI) DTG+ TDF/FTC (AI) EVG/COBI/TAF/FTC(***) EVG/COBI/TDF/FTC (AI) RAL + TDF/FTC (AI) <u>PI-based regimen</u> DRV/r + TDF/FTC (AI)	Use ABC only if HLA B*5701 negative patients Use TAF only if CrCL ≥ 30 ml/min Use EVG/COBI/TDF/FTC only if CrCL ≥70 ml/min Use TDF if CrCL ≥ 60 ml/min
Alternative Options*	**Caution**
<u>NNRTI-based regimens</u> EFV/TDF/FTC (BI) RPV/TAF/FTC(***) RPV/TDF/FTC (BI) <u>PI-based regimens</u> ATV/c + TDF/FTC(BI) ATV/r + TDF/FTC (BI) DRV/c + ABC/3TC (BIII) DRV/r + ABC/3TC (BII) DRV/c + TDF/FTC(BII)	Use RPV-based regimen only if VL <100,000 c/mL and CD4 >200/mm³ Use TAF if CrCL ≥ 30 mL/min Use TDF if CrCL ≥ 60 ml/min Use COBI only if CrCL ≥70 ml/min Use COBI only if CrCL ≥70 ml/min and ABC if HLA B*5701 negative. Use COBI only if CrCL ≥70 ml/min
Other Options**	**Caution**
<u>InSTI-based regimens</u> RAL + ABC/3TC (CII) <u>NNRTI-based regimens</u> EFV + ABC/3TC (CI) <u>PI-based regimens</u> ATV/c + ABC/3TC (CIII) ATV/r + ABC/3TC (CI) LPV/r + ABC/3TC (CI) LPV/r + ABC/3TC (CI) LPV/r + TDF/FTC (CI)	Use ABC only if HLA B*5701 negative patients Use ABC only if HLA B*5701 negative patients and pre-treatment VL <100,000 copies/mL Use ABC only if HLA B*5701 negative patients and pre-treatment VL <100,000 copies/mL
Regimen when TDF and ABC contraindicated	**Caution**
DRV/r + RAL (CI) LPV/r bid + 3TC bid (CI)	Use if pre-treatment VL <100,000 copies/mL and CD4 >200 mm³

*Alphabetical order for combinations within major categories
** When compared to preferred and alternative regimens, these regimens may have reduced virologic efficacy, limited large comparative clinical studies, or other factors (eg increased side effects, large pill burden, potential drug-drug interactions)
***Co-formulation not yet evaluated by DHHS. Added by authors based on efficacy and improved safety of TAF co-formulation.

TABLE 26: **Advantages and Disadvantages of Initial ART Regimens: Adapted from DHHS Guidelines 2016**

Drugs	Advantages	Disadvantages
Non-Nucleoside Reverse Transcriptase Inhibitors		
EFV	QD dosing; EFV/TDF/FTC coformulation; long term experience; potency with high viral load when combined with TDF/FTC.	Transmitted resistance more common than with other agents; CNS toxicity, including increased suicidality; potential teratogenicity in first 8 weeks of pregnancy; dyslipidemia; drug interaction-CYP450; empty stomach preferred
RPV	QD dosing; RPV/TDF/FTC (Complera) and RPV/TAF/FTC (Odefsey) co-formulation; small dissolvable pill. Better tolerated than EFV, including less CNS toxicity, lipid effects, and rash. RPV/TAF/FTC co-formulation may be used in patients with CrCL 30-69 mL/min.	Unlike EFV recommend only if VL <100,000 c/mL and CD4 >200/mm^3; transmitted resistance higher compared to PI-based regimen (also more common compared with InSTI regimens); gastric acid and meal requirement; CYP450 inducer and inhibitor may decrease and increase RPV levels, respectively; RPV resistance with 138K mutation results in ETR cross-resisance; QTc prolongation with increased concentrations.
Integrase Inhibitors (InSTI)		
DTG	QD dosing; superior to EFV and DRV/r due to better tolerability; higher barrier to resistance than EVG and RAL; Co-formulated DTG/ABC/3TC tablet; no food requirement; few drug-drug interactions	Decreased absorption with Al, Ca, or Mg-containing antacid and vitamins; SCr elevation (no effect on true GFR); drug interaction with UDP-glucuro- syltransferase (UGT) inducer (eg rifampin); coformulated only with ABC/3TC.
EVG/c	QD dosing; EVG/COBI/TDF/FTC (Stribild) and EVG/COBI/TAF/FTC (Genvoya) co-formulation. Lower LDL cholesterol elevation compared to ATV/r. EVG/COBI/TAF/FTC co-formulation may be used in patients with CrCL 30-69 mL/min.	Decreased absorption with Al, Ca, or Mg-containing antacid and vitamins; COBI causes SCr elevation (no effect on true GFR); Lower barrier to resistance than PI/r or DTG-based regimen; food requirement; drug interaction-metabolized via CYP3A4; ADR include H/A, transient diarrhea, nausea.
RAL	More post-marketing clinical experience than EVG/c and DTG; no food requirement; few drug-drug interactions	Decreased absorption with Al or Mg-antacid; BID dosing; low genetic barrier to resistance than PI/r and DTG-based regimen; ADR: CK elevation, myopathy, rhabdomyolysis; hypersensitivity reaction (including rare cases of TEN and SJS); drug interaction with UDP-glucurosyltransferase (UGT) inducer (eg rifampin)

(continued)

TABLE 26: Advantages and Disadvantages of Initial ART Regimens: Adapted from DHHS Guidelines 2016 (cont.)

Drugs	Advantages	Disadvantages
Protease Inhibitors		
ATV/r ATV/c	QD dosing; high resistance barrier when boosted with RTV or COBI; co-formulated with COBI	ADR: benign hyperbilirubinemia, cholethiasis, nephrotoxicity, nephrolithiasis, GI intolerance; drug interactions-CYP3A4 inhibitor; COBI boosting-avoid TDF with CrCL <70 ml/min.
DRV/r DRV/c	QD dosing; high resistance barrier; co-formulated with COBI	ADR: Rash, GI intolerance; food requirement; drug interactions-CYP3A4 inhibitor; DRV/c: less clinical experience and unable to co-administer with NNRTIs; COBI boosting avoid TDF with CrCL < 70 ml/min
LPV/r	No food requirement; co-formulation; Dosing QD or BID	Requires 200mg/d RTV; ADR-possible MI risk; PR and QT prolongation; possible nephrotoxicity, also more GI toxicity; drug interactions-CYP3A4 inhibitor
Dual-NRTI		
ABC/3TC	Co-formulated DTG/ABC/3TC tablet Good potency with VL >100,000 c/mL when given with DTG	Inferior virologic response w/ VL >100,0000 c/mL when combined with ATV/r or EFV; severe hypersensitivity reaction in HLA B*5701 positive patients; associated with increased risk of MI in some studies (debated issue despite extensive data)
TAF/FTC	Co-formulated EVG/COBI/TAF/FTC and RPV/TAF/FTC tablets. Lower rates of nephrotoxicity and BMD loss compared to TDF/FTC No dose adjustment for CrCL >30 ml/min	Not recommended for HBV treatment Not recommended for PrEP Avoid TAF with CrCL < 30 ml/min No long-term data
TDF/FTC	Co-formulated EFV/TDF/FTC, EVG/COBI/TDF/FTC, RPV/TDF/FTC tablets; active against HBV; better virologic response at baseline VL > 100,000 c/mL than ABC/3TC when combined with EFV or ATV/r	Nephrotoxicity-proximal tubular dysfunction with acute and chronic renal insufficiency; nephrotoxicity risk may be increased with COBI or RTV-boosted PI administration. Avoid TDF with CrCL < 60 ml/min

TABLE 27: Factors affecting initial ART selection (DHHS guidelines 2016)

Factor	Recommendation	Concern or alternative
CD4 <200 cells/mm³	• Avoid RPV-based regimen • Avoid DRV/r+RAL	Increased rate of virologic failure
VL >100,000 c/mL	• Avoid RPV-based regimen and DRV/r+RAL • Avoid ABC/3TC combined with ATV/r or EFV	Increased rate of virologic failure
HLA B*5701 positive	• Avoid ABC	High risk of severe ABC hypersensitivity reaction
No baseline resistance tests available	• Avoid NNRTI-based regimen • Use PI/r-based regimen	Transmission of NNRTI resistant virus more likely than PI/r or InSTI If NRTI resistance suspected based on ARV history, some experts recommend avoiding INSTI-based regimen.
Convenience of one pill once daily	Fixed dose combination: •DTG/ABC/3TC (Triumeq) •EFV/TDF/FTC (Atripla) •EVG/COBI/TDF/FTC (Stribild) and EVG/COBI/TAF/FTC (Genvoya) RPV/TDF/FTC (Complera) and RPV/TAF/FTC (Odefsey)	Use EVG/COBI/TAF/FTC and RPV/TAF/FTC only if CrCL >30 mL/min Use EVG/COBI/TDF/FTC only if CrCL >70 ml/min. Use RPV/TAF/FTC or RPV/TDF/FTC only if VL <100,000 c/mL an CD4 count > 200 cells/mm3
Food effects	Must take with food: •RPV-based regimen •ATV/r and ATV/c •DRV/r and DRV/c •EVG/COBI/TDF/FTC *EVG/COBI/TAF/FTC Take on empty stomach: EFV	Food improves absorption Food increases EFV absorption and may increase CNS side effect (esp during the first 2 weeks). Can be taken with food if tolerated.
Renal disease	Consider avoiding TDF If eGFR <70 ml/min: avoid EVG/COBI/TDF/FTC ATV/c + TDF/FTC DRV/c +TDF/FTC If eGFR < 60 ml/min: avoid ABC/3TC co-formulation If CrCL <30 ml/min, avoid TAF/FTC, EVG/COBI/TAF/FTC, and RPV/TAF/FTC	ABC-based regimen or DRV/r+RAL can be considered instead of TDF. If TDF used with CKD, modify TDF dose Use standard dose ABC and dose adjusted 3TC
Osteoporosis/ osteopenia	Avoid TDF	TDF may decrease bone mineral density with renal tubulopathy, urine phosphate wasting, and osteomalacia Consider TAF or ABC

TABLE 27: Factors affecting initial ART selection (DHHS guidelines 2016) *(cont.)*

Factor	Recommendation	Comment
Psychiatric illness or HIV dementia or methadone maintenance	Consider avoiding EFV	EFV may exacerbate psychiatric symptoms and confound assessment of HIV dementia improvement on ART. Methadone levels may significantly decrease with EFV co-administration. Methadone dose may need to be increased to prevent withdrawal symptoms
High cardiac risk	Consider avoiding ABC- and LPV/r-based regimen	Increased cardiovascular risk inconsistently shown in large cohort studies.
Hyperlipidemia	PI/r, (less with ATV/r and DRV/r)ABC, EFV, and EVG/c have been associated with increased serum lipids	Consider alternative ART
Pregnancy	Consider ATV/r, LPV/r, EFV (after 8 weeks gestation) PLUS ABC/3TC, TDF/FFTC, or AZT/3TC.	Stay on current ARV regimen if VL <50 c/mL See pregnancy section page 69
HBV infection	Use TDF/FTC (or TDF + 3TC) If TDF cannot be used: Entecavir + FTC or 3TC for HBV treatment	TDF, FTC, and 3TC are active against HBV TAF active against HBV, but not FDA approved for HBV. Use two active agents to prevent the rapid emergence of lamivudine resistant HBV. Severe HBV flare associated with TDF/FTC or TAF/FTC discontinuation with HBV-HIV co-infection
HCV infection	Ledipasvir-Sofobuvir: use TDF with renal function monitoring when combined with PI/r or EFV or use TAF Simepravir-SOF: use RAL+TDF/FTC or RAL+TAF/FTC Dasabuvir, ombitasvir, paritaprevir, RTV: Can use ATV 300mg/d or possibly DTG or RAL	See table 17 for HCV drug interactions Minimal drug ARV interactions with ledipasvir-sofosbuvir regimen. Simepravir: avoid PIs, NNRTIs (except RPV)
TB co-infection	With rifampin co-administration: Use EFV 600 mg/d, RAL 800 mg BID, or DTG 50 mg BID (in pts without select INSTI mutations defined in DTG package insert) If PI/r-based regimen needed: use rifabutin (dose 150mg/d or 300mg 3x/week)	PI/r co-administration with rifampin contraindicated TAF not recommended with rifampin, rifabutin, and rifapentine. Monitor rifabutin levels

TABLE 28: **Methods to Achieve Readiness to Start ART and Maintain Adherence**

Patient-related methods
• Negotiate a plan or regimen that the patient understands and to which she/he commits • Consider patient preferences: pill burden (frequency) and pill size, food effect, drug interactions • Recruit family, friends, peer, and community support • Use memory aids: timers, pagers, written schedule, pill boxes/medication organizers • Plan ahead: keep extra meds in key locations, obtain refills • Use missed doses as opportunities to prevent future misses • Address financial issues: copays, insurance, etc. • Active drug and alcohol use and mental illness predict poor adherence; race, sex, age, educational level, income, and *past* drug use do not
Provider- /Health team-related
• Educate patient re: goals of therapy, pills, food effects, and side effects • Assess adherence potential before ART; monitor at each visit • Ensure access at off-hours and weekends for questions or addressing problems • Utilize full health care team; ensure med refills at pharmacy • Consider impact of new diagnoses, intercurrent illness and events on adherence • Provide training updates on adherence for all team members and utilize team to reinforce adherence • Monitor adherence and intensify management in periods of low adherence • Educate volunteers, patient-community representatives • Treat mental illness (e.g., depression) and substance abuse
Regimen-related
• Avoid adverse drug interactions • Simplify regimen re: dosing frequency, pill burden, and food requirements when feasible • Inform patient about anticipated side effects • Anticipate and treat side effects
Monitoring adherence
• Viral load – expect a decrease of 1-2 $\log_{10}$ c/mL by 4 weeks, VL < 400 c/mL by 8-16 weeks and then sustained levels < 20 c/mL: Documenting viral suppression is the most important metric for monitoring adherence since recommended regimens virtually always work (unless there is an unforeseen drug interaction or undetected baseline resistance). Note that viral suppression is the primary goal of treatment. • Pill counts and pharmacy records are useful for documenting adherence

TABLE 29: Management of ART Treatment Failure

Virologic Failure

- **Definition:** Goal is to acheive VL < 20-75 c/mL by 24 weeks. The expected VL response to ART is a 0.75-1.0 $\log_{10}$ c/mL by 1 week, 1.5-2.0 $\log_{10}$ by 4 weeks, VL <5,000 c/mL at 8-16 weeks and < 20 c/mL at 24-48 weeks.
- **Virologic failure:** Two consecutive HIV RNA levels > 200 c/mL after 24 weeks of ART
- **Blip:** Isolated detectable HIV RNA level (200-400 c/mL) followed by return to suppression to <200 c/mL
- **Causes:** Resistance (transmitted or acquired), usually reflects non-adherence; drug-drug interactions less common
- **Resistance test:** Preferably done during ART or within 4 weeks of stopping ART. Requires VL of >500-1000 c/mL. Cost: genotype $300-400; Phenotype: $800-1200
- Boosted PIs (DRV/r; ATV/r; LPV/r) all have a high genetic barrier to resistance. Thus, most patients with viral failure on PI/r-based ART who fail will have sensitive strains of HIV unless the drug is continued with viral failure for prolonged periods. DTG also appears to have a higher barrier to resistance compared to RAL and EVG. Resistance to other antiretrovirals (esp NNRTIs, 3TC, FTC) occurs more rapidly when there is virologic failure.
- **Resistance resources:**Stanford University HIV database: http://hivdb.stanford.edu; IAS-USA: http://iasusa.org
- **Goal:** Always use at least two drugs in two classes that are active *in vitro*, and preferably three active agents.
- **Admonitions:** Never add a single agent to a failing regimen; 2) Do not stop ART since this will lead to rapid increase in VL and rapid decrease in CD4 count, with potential for resistance, especially with NNRTI-based regimens.

Resistance Tests (see Table 31 Indications for Resistance Testing)

- Usually genotypic test, especially with early sequence failure.
- Testing should be done during therapy or within 4 wks of cessation of the failed regimen, if possible.
- Need for separate (or combined) InSTI genotype in patients failing InSTI-based regimens.
- A viral load of > 500-1,000 c/mL is usually required for the currently available resistance tests, but GenoSure Archive in patients with low or undetectable VL.
- Virologic failure of recommended first-line regimens are generally due to transmitted resistance or poor adherence.
- Phenotypic resistance assay can augment genotypic resistance tests in patients with multiple resistance mutations after multiple virologic failures. Especially useful in cases of complex PI resistance.

Using Resistance Test Results

- Interpretation of resistance tests results is complex and sometimes requires expert consultation.
- Interpretation should include the history of prior antiretroviral treatments and results of prior resistance tests. Past resistance mutations, even if not detected on the most recent test, remain relevant.
- Failure to detect resistance mutations in the presence of failed treatment usually indicates non-adherence.
- Resistance tests are best for indicating drugs or drug classes that will not work rather than those that will work.

Immunologic Failure

- Failure to increase CD4 count 25-50/mm³ during first year.
- Mean increase is about 100-150/mm³ in first year with ART in treatment naive patients who achieve viral suppression; at 3-5 years the increase averages 20-50/mm³/year.
- No data support switching ARVs when viral load is undetectable to improve CD4 response except for ADRs.
- Long term studies show that half of patients who start ART with a CD4 < 100/mm³ never achieve a CD4 count > 500/mm³. Attempts to improve CD4 response with methods other than viral suppression have been generally unsuccessful.

Clinical Failure

Occurrence or recurrence of HIV-related event reflecting HIV viremia ≥ 3 months after start of ART.
Note: Must exclude immune reconstitution syndromes (IRIS).

TABLE 30: **Management of Treatment Experienced Patients (DHHS Guidelines Jan. 28, 2016)**

Expert Advice: Should be sought
Evaluation: assess adherence, drug-drug interactions, drug food interactions, drug tolerance; HIV VL and CD4 count history; treatment history; prior and recent resistance test results
Resistance testing: Test during ART or within 4 weeks of stopping ART. Later testing still may be useful since resistance mutations may be detected.
New Regimen: Should include 2 or preferably 3 active agents
Virologic suppression not possible: Continue ART to maximize anti-HIV activity and minimize toxicity
Discontinue ART: Likely to result in rapid increase in VL and decrease CD4 count- Not recommended

TABLE 31: **Indications for Resistance Testing**

Indicated
• Virologic failure with VL > 500-1,000 c/mL • Acute HIV infection • Baseline, (entry to care) prior to initial therapy
Not Indicated
• After discontinuation of antiretroviral therapy > 1 month duration. Positive results are helpful, but negative results do not exclude resistance mutations. • With VL <1,000 c/mL, consider GenoSure Archive.

TABLE 32: Resistance Mutations (*Top HIV Med*, 2014; 22: 642)

Drug	Codon Mutations
Nucleosides and Nucleotides - Reverse Transcriptase Mutations	
3TC	65R,184VI
ABC	65R/E/N, 74V, 115F, 184V
AZT[1]	41L, 67N, 70R, 210W, 215Y/F, 219Q/E
d4T[1]	41L, 65R/E/N, 67N, 70R, 210W, 215Y/F, 219Q/E
ddI	65R/E/N, 74V
FTC	65R/E/N, 184V/I
TAF and TDF[1]	65R/E/N, 70E
Multi-nRTI resistance (TAMs)	41L, 67N, 70R, 210W, 215Y/F, 219Q/E
Multinucleoside Q151M plus	62V, 75I, 77L, 116Y, 151M
Multinucleoside 69 Insertion	41L, 62V, 69 insert, 70R, 210W, 215Y/F, 219Q/E
Non-Nucleoside Reverse Transcriptase Inhibitors	
EFV	100I, 101P, 103N/S, 106M, 108I, 181C/I, 188L, 190S/A, 225H, 230L
ETR[2*]	90I, 98G, 100I, 101E/H/P, 106I, 138A/G/K/Q, 179D/F/T, 181C/I/V, 190S/A, 230L
NVP	100I, 101P, 103N/S, 106A/M, 108I, 181C/I, 188C/L/H, 190A, 230L
RPV	100I, 101E/P, 138AGKQR, 179L, 181C/L/V, 188L, 221Y, 227C, 230I/L

1 TAMs (induced by AZT or d4T) counteract selection of 65R
2 ETR: Most resistance requires 181C plus ≥ 3 baseline mutations to show reduced response.
* Tibotec Scoring System, weighted scoring system (based on DUET studies, HIV Med 2012; 13:427)
- 3 points: 181I/V; • 2.5 points: 101P, 100I, 181C, 230L; • 1.5 points: 90I, 138A, 190S, 179F; • 1 point: 179D, 179T, 101E, 101H, 98G, 190A:
  0-2 points: susceptible; 2.5-3.5 points: intermediate resistance; 4+ points: high level resistance

TABLE 32: **Resistance Mutations** *(cont.)*

Drug	Major**	Minor**
Protease Inhibitors - Protease Gene Mutations		
FPV/r	50V, 84V	10FIRV, 32I, 46IL, 47V, 54LVM, 73S, 76V, 82AFST, 90M
ATV[3]	50L, 84V, 88S	10IFVC, 16E, 20RMITV, 24I, 32I, 33IFV, 34Q, 36ILV, 46IL, 48V, 53LY, 54LVMTA, 60E, 62V, 64LMV, 71VITL, 73CSTA, 82ATFI, 85V, 90M, 93LM
DRV[8]	47V, 50V, 54ML, 76V, 84V	11I, 32I, 33F, 74P, 89V
IDV/r	46I/L, 82AFT, 84V	10IRV, 20MR, 24I, 32I, 36I, 54V, 71VT, 73SA, 76V, 77I, 90M
LPV/r[4]	32I, 47VA, 76V, 82AFTS	10FIRV, 20MR, 24I, 33F, 46IL, 50V, 53L, 54VLAMTS, 63P, 71VT, 73S, 84V, 90M
NFV	30N, 90M	10FI, 36I, 46IL, 71VT, 77I, 82AFTS, 84V, 88DS
SQV/r	48V, 90M	10IRV, 24I, 54VL, 62V, 71VT, 73S, 77I, 82AFTS, 84V
TPV/r[5]	47V, 58E, 74P, 82LT, 83D, 84V	10V, 33F, 36ILV, 43T, 46L, 54AMV, 69KR, 89IMV
Entry Inhibitors		
T-20	gp41 envelope -- 36DS, 37V, 38AME, 39R, 40H, 42T, 43D	
MVC[6]	X4 virus, dual or mixed tropic virus. Also mutations on HIV-1 gp120 V3 loop	
Integrase Inhibitors - Integrase Mutations		**Comment**
DTG[9]	121Y, 138A/K, 140S/A, 148H	May retain activity in some RAL and EVG resistant virus.
EVG	66I/A/K, 92Q/G, 97A, 121Y, 147G, 148R/H/K, 155H	The sequential use of EVG and RAL is not recommended due to the potential of cross-resistance.
RAL[7]	74M, 92Q, 97A, 121Y, 138A/K, 155H, 143R/H/C, 148H/K/R, 155H	The sequential use of EVG and RAL is not recommended due to potential of cross-resistance

** Major mutations usually develop first and are usually associated with decreased drug binding; Minor mutations also contribute to drug resistance; may affect drug binding in vitro less than primary mutations. Use of Major and Minor designations for NRTIs and NNRTIs has been suspended.

3 ATV: ≥ 3 of the following mutations reduce viral response: 10FIV, 16E, 33FIV, 46IL, 60E, 84V, 85V. Another report implicates ≥ 3 of the following 10CV, 32I, 34Q, 46IL, 53L, 54AMV, 82FV, 84V.

4 LPV: ≥ 6 mutations required for resistance: 47A (and possibly 47V and 32I impart high level resistance.

5 TPV: ≥ 2 of the following mutations correlates with reduced response: 33G, 82IT, 84V, and 90M.

6 MVC: X4, mixed or dual tropic virus does not respond to MVC. Some mutations at codon 4, 11 and 19 of the V3 loop appear important but are not well defined and testing from commercial sources is not available. Emergence of X4 virus is more important.

7 RAL: Two major pathways: 148HKR or 155H with minor mutation. For 148HKR these are 74M, 38A1, 138K, or 140S. The most common and most potent cause of lost sensitivity is 148H and 140S. For 155H pathway the additional primary mutations are 74M, 92Q, 97A, 143H, 163KR, 151I, or 232N.

8 With 0-2, 3, or ≥ 4 of 47V, 54M, 74P & 84V DRV mutations at baseline, the virologic response (< 500 c/mL at 24 weeks) was 50%, 22%, and 10% respectively.

9 DTG: Q148H and G140S w/ mutations 74I/M, 92Q,97A, 138A/K, 140A, 155H associated with DTG resistance

TABLE 33: Indications for ART: WHO Guidelines for Resource-limited Settings June 2013*

When to start	
All Patients with CD4 ≤ 500 cells/mm³ HIGH PRIORITY: WHO clinical stage 3 or 4 irrespective of CD4 count.; count ≤ 350 cells/mm³	
All patients with active TB regardless of CD4 count	
HBV/HIV co-infection with severe chronic liver disease requiring HBV treatment	
ARVs should be offered to decrease transmission to HIV-negative partner	
All pregnant and breastfeeding women	
Clinical Stages	
Clinical Stage 1	Asymptomatic or PGL, and/or normal activity
Clinical Stage 2	Weight loss < 10%, minor mucocutaneous conditions, zoster < 5 years, recurrent URIs, and/or symptomatic plus normal activity
Clinical Stage 3	Weight loss > 10%, unexplained diarrhea > 1 mo, unexplained fever > 1 mo, thrush, oral hairy leukoplakia, pulmonary TB in past year, or severe bacterial infection, and/or bedridden < 50% of days in the past month
Clinical Stage 4	CDC-defined AIDS and/or bedridden > 50% of days in the past month

TABLE 34: Starting Regimens for Antiretroviral Naive Patients: WHO Guidelines for Resource-limited Settings June 2013

Patient Criteria	Regimen
ARV-naive	Preferred: TDF+3TC (or FTC) PLUS EFV Alternative: AZT/3TC/EFV (OR NVP); TDF/3TC (or FTC)/NVP
TB co-infection	Preferred: TDF/3TC/EFV (with rifampin) Start ART as soon as possible (within 8 weeks of anti-TB treatment) Start ART immediately w/anti-TB drugs if CD4 < 50

"Special circumstances": regimen with ABC, d4T, and PI/r.

TABLE 35: **When to Change ART Regimens: WHO Guidelines for Resource-limited Settings June 2013**

Failure	Definition
Clinical	New or recurrent stage 4 condition (Table 33). Exceptions are lymph node or pleural TB, candida esophagitis, and recurrent bacterial pneumonia; must rule-out IRIS
CD4 count	Fall to baseline level; 50% fall from treatment peak; or levels persistently < 100 cells/mm^3
Virologic	VL > 5,000 c/mL. This level is associated with clinical progression and rapid CD4 decline
-*Viral load is recommended as the preferred monitoring approach to diagnose and confirm ARV treatment failure* -*If viral load is not routinely available, CD4 count and clinical monitoring should be used to diagnose treatment failure* -*Clinical disease progression:* events occurring > 6 mos after starting ARV because events in the first 6 mos often represent IRIS. New or recurrent events in the first 6 mos meriting change in therapy are AIDS-defining conditions (WHO clinical stage 4). Consider changing therapy for these WHO clinical stage 3 conditions: weight loss > 10%, unexplained diarrhea or fever > 1 mo, oral hairy leukoplakia, severe bacterial infection, or bedridden > 50% of days in past month	

TABLE 36: **What ART Regimen to Change to: WHO Guidelines for Resource-limited Settings June 2013**

Initial Regimen Included	Second Line Becomes
(NVP or EFV) + the below pairings:	PI/r: Heat stable fixed dose combination (LPV/r, ATV/r)
• (AZT or d4T) + 3TC†	TDF + (3TC ±AZT)‡ + (ATV/r or LPV/r)
• TDF + (3TC or FTC)†	AZT + (3TC or FTC) + (ATV/r or LPV/r)

† 3TC and FTC are considered interchangeable; they are structurally related and share pharmacological properties and resistance profiles.

‡ 3TC can be maintained in second line regimens to potentially reduce viral fitness, confer residual antiviral activity, and maintain pressure on the M184V mutation to improve viral sensitivity to AZT or TDF. AZT continuation may prevent or delay emergence of the K65R mutation, but continuation leads to TAMs and cross resistance to all NRTIs.

PREGNANCY AND HIV (DHHS Pregnancy Perinatal Guidelines August 6, 2015)

Hot Line: The National Perinatal HIV Hotline (1-888-448-8765) provides free consultative service for all aspects of perinatal HIV care.

HIV testing: All pregnant women should be tested (with 4th generation HIV test) at entry to care; repeat if symptoms of acute retroviral syndrome (acute HIV).

Registry: All cases of ART exposure during pregnancy-report to Antiretroviral Pregnancy Registry (http://www.apregistry.com)

EFV: Non-pregnant with childbearing potential should have pregnancy testing before receiving EFV and receive counseling on this toxicity. The risk of neural tube defects (due to EFV) is limited to the first 5-6 weeks of gestation and pregnancy is rarely recognized that early; thus, can be continued in pregnancy after the first trimester.

ART: All pregnant women with HIV infection should receive ART to prevent perinatal transmission regardless of baseline CD4 count or viral load.

-Initiate ART as soon as HIV is diagnosed during pregnancy.

-Resistance testing should be done before starting ART, but ART should be started without waiting for resistance test results with advanced HIV infection or late in pregnancy when ART should be started empirically.

-Urgency here is defined by CD4 count, viral load, and maternal conditions (nausea and vomiting)

Drug selection-ART-naive

Use DHHS guidelines for drug selection with appropriate attention to baseline resistance test results, comorbidities, convenience, adverse reactions, drug interactions, experience with use in pregnancy and risk of teratogenicity. Risk of delaying to gestation week 12 depends on CD4 count and drug tolerance.

Favored Regimens (see Table 37): ABC/3TC or TDF/FTC PLUS PI/r (ATV/r or DRV/r) OR EFV (if after 8 week gestation) OR RAL

Drug selection: ART Experienced: Continue regimen (including EFV) if viral suppression achieved and regimen is tolerated.

Risk reduction counseling: Women with HIV infected partners should be alerted to the high risk of HIV transmission to the neonate during acute HIV infection. PrEP should be considered.

Amniocentesis: Should only be done with VL < 50 c/mL at the time of the procedure.

PREGNANCY AND HIV (DHHS Pregnancy Perinatal Guidelines August 6, 2016)

C-section: Pregnant women with suboptimal HIV suppression should be counseled on benefit of C-section to be performed at 38 weeks gestation.
Requirements:

1) VL consistently > 1000 c/mL in late pregnancy
2) Last viral load was obtained within 4 weeks of delivery
3) Patient has been adherent to ART and confirms no missed ARV doses in past 4 weeks

Note:

1) It is unclear if C-section to prevent mother to child transmission (MTCT) if done after onset of labor or rupture of membranes.
2) Oxytocin suggested when prolonged labor after rupture of membranes.
3) C-section has not been proven to reduce MTCT if a) Maternal VL <1,000 c/mL b) Membrane rupture over 4 hours c) Patient is in active labor

Intra-partum care:
-If possible, avoid artificial rupture of membranes, use of fetal scalp electrodes, and delivery with foreceps, vacuum extractor, and episiotomy.
-Continue ART as much as possible during labor and before scheduled C-section. If HIV VL > 1,000 c/mL or unknown-give IV AZT near delivery and schedule C-section. C-section is unnecessary for women with consistent HIV suppression (VL <1,000 c/mL) in late pregnancy.

Infant ART: Initiate AZT for 6 wks starting within 6-12 hrs after delivery

Untreated Mother during pregnancy: AZT x 6 wks plus NVP at birth, 48hrs and 144 hrs

Maternal HIV status unknown: Rapid HIV test of mother or infant and immediate AZT for infant

Breast-feeding: This should be avoided until HIV is excluded.

TABLE 37: Antiretroviral Drugs in Pregnancy (2015 NY State AIDS guidelines and DHHS Pregnancy and Perinatal Guidelines August 6, 2015)

Advisory	Drugs
Nucleosides and Nucleotides	
Recommended	ABC/3TC; AZT/3TC; TDF/FTC** or 3TC (standard doses)
Not recommended	ddI; d4T; ddI/d4T (contraindicated); ABC/3TC/ZDV
Non-nucleoside RT Inhibitors	
Recommended	EFV* (initiate after first 8 weeks of pregnancy)
Alternative Regimen	RPV* (avoid in VL >100K or CD4 <200 cells/mm3)
Not recommended	NVP (Avoid in women with baseline CD4 > 250 cells/mm^3; monitor for HSR) ETR (not recommended in ARV-naive pts)
Protease Inhibitors	
Recommended	ATV/r* 300/100 mg once-daily DRV/r* 600/100 mg bid (avoid once-daily dosing)
Alternatives	LPV/r* 2 or 3 tabs bid in third trimester (avoid once-daily dosing in pregnancy).
Insufficient data to recommend	FPV
Not recommended	NFV (low efficacy), TPV (not recommended in ARV-naive pts), IDV/r (nephrolithiasis), high dose RTV (high toxicity and low efficacy); SQV/r (must get baseline ECG. Not recommended if QTc and/or PR prolongation).
Entry Inhibitors	
Insufficient data to recommend	MVC
Not recommended	ENF (not recommended in ART-naive pts)
Integrase Inhibitors	
Preferred	RAL*
Insufficient data to recommend	DTG; EVG+COBI

* Combine with preferred two-NRTI backbone
** Preferred NRTI in HBV co-infected patients

TABLE 38: **Recommendations for Clinical Scenarios (2015 NY State AIDS guidelines and DHHS Pregnancy Perinatal Guidelines August 6, 2015)**

<table>
<tr><th>Clinical Setting</th><th colspan="2">Recommendation</th></tr>
<tr><td>Pregnancy potential plus indications for ART</td><td colspan="2">Initiate ART per DHHS guidelines; avoid EFV unless contraception adequate. Exclude pregnancy before starting EFV</td></tr>
<tr><td>Receiving ART; becomes pregnant</td><td colspan="2">1. Continue ART if viral suppression achieved even if EFV-based regimen
2. Labor: Continue HAART po and give IV AZT at delivery† if VL >1000 copies/mL
3. Schedule C-Section at 38 wks if VL > 1,000 c/mL near delivery
4. AZT for infant x 6 wks§ plus 3 doses of NVP 2mg/kg (first dose at birth to 48 hours,second dose 48 hours after first dose, and third dose 96 hours after second dose) in the first week of life for infants born to mothers who did not receive antepartum ARV drugs or received only intrapartum drugs</td></tr>
<tr><td>Treatment-naive, indications for ART and pregnant</td><td colspan="2">1. Initiate ART; ABC/3TC, TDF/FTC <u>PLUS</u> EFV (after first 8 weeks gestation), ATV/r, DRV/r, or RAL
2. Follow 2-4 above</td></tr>
<tr><td>Treatment-naive, CD4 > 500/mm^3 and pregnant</td><td colspan="2">1. Initiate ART (regimen above) to prevent perinatal transmission
2. Follow 2-4 above
3. Evaluate feasibility of continuing ART post-partum. If plan is to discontinue NNRTI-based ART: Continue 2 NRTIs 7d after stopping NNRTI</td></tr>
<tr><td>Prior ART, now off treatment and pregnant</td><td colspan="2">1. Initiate ART based on history and current and prior resistance test results
2. Follow 2-4 above</td></tr>
<tr><td>Acute HIV in pregnancy</td><td colspan="2">1. Risk of transmission to fetus is very high due to viral load often > 1 million/mL
2. Rapid testing (4th generation test) and institution of ART indicated.</td></tr>
<tr><td rowspan="3">Treatment-naive and presents in labor</td><td colspan="2">Options</td></tr>
<tr><td>Mother</td><td>Infant</td></tr>
<tr><td>AZT IV† during labor
+ NVP 200 mg po x1
+ AZT/3TC x7d po post-partum.
Evaluate feasibility for ART</td><td>AZT§ x 6wks plus 3 doses of NVP in the first week of life for infants born</td></tr>
<tr><td>Untreated HIV+ mother with newborn infant</td><td colspan="2">Infant: AZT x 6 wks plus 3 doses of NVP in the first week of life for newborn infants
Mother: Evaluate feasibility of ART</td></tr>
</table>

† AZT intrapartum: 2 mg/kg/h x 1h, then 1 mg/kg/h until delivery

§ AZT for infant < 35 weeks gestation: 1.5 mg/kg IV q12h or 2 mg/kg po q12h, increasing to q8h at 2 weeks if > 30 weeks gestation at birth or at 4 weeks if < 30 weeks gestation at birth AZT x 4 weeks can be considered if mother had an undetectable viral load throughout pregnancy.

TABLE 39: Antiretrovirals Data and Concerns for Pregnancy

Agent	Human Studies in Pregnancy	Concerns
	Nucleoside and Nucleotide Reverse Transcriptase Inhibitors	
3TC	Well tolerated, Good pharmacokinetics with high placental transfer to fetus; not teratogenic	If mother's HBV co-infected, possible HBV flare with discontinuation.
ABC	Good pharmacokinetics at standard doses w/high placental transfer to fetus; not teratogenic	Must screen for HLA-B*5701
AZT	Good pharmacokinetics w/ high placental transfer to fetus. Extensive studies showing efficacy in reducing MTCT	Bone marrow suppression and poor GI tolerance
d4T	Good pharmacokinetics w/ high placental transfer to fetus; not teratogenic.	Lactic acidosis, especially when combined with ddl
ddl	Good pharmacokinetics with low to moderate placental transfer to fetus; increased risk of birth defects	Lactic acidosis rates increased, especially when combined with d4T
FTC	Slightly lower level in 3rd trimester; use standard dose; high placental transfer to fetus; not teratogenic.	If HBV co-infected, possible HBV flare with discontinuation.
TDF	Lower AUC in 3rd trimester, but trough adequate; high placental transfer to fetus; not teratogenic Preferred if HBV-co-infected	Primate study shows reduced fetal bone porosity, Human studies showed no effect on intrauterine growth. Conflicting data about potential effects on growth outcome later in pregnancy. If HBV co-infected, possible HBV flare with discontinuation. Monitor renal function. PROMISE (CROI 2015) showed higher infant deaths (0.6% vs. 4.4%) than with AZT.
	Non- Nucleoside Reverse Transcriptase Inhibitors	
EFV	Teratogenic in primates study. Avoid in the first 8 weeks of pregnancy or pregnancy vulnerable due to inadequate contraception AUC decreased during 3rd trimester, but trough adequate in nearly all patients w/ moderate placental transfer to fetus.	Risk of neural tube defect in first 8 weeks of gestation. FDA pregnancy category D, but if VL <50 c/mLswitching off EFV not recommended due to risk of loss of viral control and increased risk of perinatal transmission.
NVP	Good pharmacokinetics with high placental transfer to the fetus, safety and efficacy of single perinatal dose to prevent transmission shown in many trials. Not teratogenic	No longer recommended as an alternative ART in pregnancy. Concern is HSR/rash treatment naive patients with baseline CD4 count > 250 cells/mm^3
RPV	Concentrations decreased 20-30% compared to post-partum. Moderate to high placental transfer to fetus	Insufficient data to recommend routine use
ETR	Concentrations increased by 20-60% in pregnancy. Not teratogenic in animal studies. Variable placental transfer (19% to 325% maternal serum concentration).	Not recommended in treatment-naive patients
	Entry Inhibitor	
ENF	No PK data. Low placental transfer to fetus	Insufficient data to recommend routine use
MVC	Limited PK data. Low placental transfer to fetus. No data on human teratogenicity.	Insufficient data to recommend routine use

TABLE 39: Antiretrovirals Data and Concerns for Pregnancy *(cont.)*

Agent	Human Studies in Pregnancy	Concerns
	Protease Inhibitors	
PI Class	Diabetes, GI intolerance	Risk of diabetes and ketoacidosis; unclear if rate is increased in pregnancy
ATV	2/3 PK studies showed decreased concentration in the third trimester w/ low placental transfer to fetus. Not teratogenic Use ATV/r 400/100 with TDF or H2 blocker coadministration in ARV-experienced patient; some experts recommend ATV/r 400/100 in all women	Hyperbilirubinemia. Non-pathologic elevations of neonatal hyperbilirubinemia in some, but not all clinical trials. Preferred PI in combination with TDF/FTC or ABC/3TC in pregnancy
DRV/r	Decreased exposure in pregnancy w/ low placental transfer to fetus. Not teratogenic in animal studies, but limited human data.	Preferred PI when used in combination with TDF/FTC or ABC/3TC in pregnancy
FPV	AUC decreased 36% in 3rd trimester, but trough higher compared to non-boosted FPV. Low placental transfer to fetus Use FPV/r 700/100 bid	Safety in pregnancy data are insufficient to recommend use during pregnancy. With FPV/r, trough adequate in PI-naive patients
IDV	AUC decreased 50-80% in pregnancy w/ minimal placental transfer to fetus. Not teratogenic	Concern for hyperbilirubinemia, but low placental transfer to fetus mitigates this concern. Not recommended in pregnancy.
LPV/r	Decreased concentrations in 2nd and 3rd trimester w/ low placental transfer to fetus. Increase dose to LPV/r 600/150 mg bid in 2nd and 3rd trimester.	Once-daily dosing not recommended in pregnancy. Avoid oral solution in pregnancy due to alcohol and propylene glycol content. LPV/r can be used as an alternative PI/r.
NFV	PACTG 353 showed doses of 1250 mg bid achieved therapeutic levels (but not 750 mg tid). Minimal to low placental transfer to fetus. Not teratogenic.	Avoid use due to lower potency compared to LPV/r
SQV	Studies with unboosted Fortovase showed reduced levels in pregnancy; data for Invirase are limited. Low placental transfer to fetus. Not teratogenic in animal studies, but limited human data. Use SQV/r 1000/100 bid	Monitor PR and QTc interval. SQV/r is no longer recommended as an alternative PI/r.
RTV	Lower concentrations in pregnancy, but no dose adjustment needed. Not teratogenic. Low placental transfer to fetus.	Avoid oral solution in pregnancy due to alcohol content.
TPV	Limited PK data. Not teratogenic in animal studies, but limited human data.	Hepatitis; Avoid
	Integrase Inhibitor	
DTG	No PK data. Not teratogenic in animal studies, but limited human data. Unknown placental transfer	Insufficient data to recommend routine use
EVG	No PK data. Not teratogenic in animal studies, but limited human data. Unknown placental transfer	Insufficient data to recommend routine use
RAL	Limited PK data suggest no change in pregnancy. Not teratogenic in rabbit studies, but limited human data. High placental transfer	Is the preferred InSTI during pregnancy when combined with TDF/FTC or ABC/3TC.

TABLE 40: **Mode of Delivery**

Clinical Setting	Recommendation
HIV infected presents at > 36 weeks, on no ART, labs pending	1. Start ART per Table 38 2. Recommend C-section at 38 weeks 3. IV AZT 3 h pre-op and single dose to infant 4. Use prophylactic antibacterials 5. Evaluate for HAART post-partum
HIV treated, pregnant and VL > 1000 c/mL at 36 weeks	1. Continue ART if VL decreasing or change if poor virologic response 2. Schedule C-section if VL likely to be > 1000 c/mL at 38 weeks 3. Continue ARV through surgical period 4. Prophylactic antibacterials for the C-section 5. Continue ART 6. Infant should receive AZT as above
Mother receiving ART with virologic control (VL <1000 c/ml	Risk of perinatal transmission is < 2%; C-section is not routinely recommended.
Mother has scheduled C-section but presents in labor	1. Give IV AZT to mother 2. Risk and benefit of C-section should be evaluated on a cases by case basis 3. Give post-partum AZT to infant

TABLE 41: **Drugs to Avoid During Pregnancy**

Agent	Class*	Recommendation
ACE Inhibitors and ARBs	D	Use alternative antihypertensive (methyldopa)
Warfarin	X	Consider heparin or LMW heparin
Anticonvulsants: carbamazapine, valproic acid, phenytoin, and phenobarbital	D	Can be continued if indicated. Consider alternate anticonvulsants.
HMG-CoA reductase inhibitor	D	Consider alternative (eg fibrinic acid, niacin)
Paroxetine	D	Consider alternative antidepressant
Miscellaneous: ergotamine, thalidomide, raloxifene, misoprostol retinoids, and benzodiazepines	X	Contraindicated
ribavirin	X	Contraindicated

* **FDA pregnancy category:**
A controlled studies show no risk
B no evidence of risk in humans
C risk not ruled out
D positive evidence of risk
X contraindicated in pregnancy

TABLE 42: **Drugs for Opportunistic Infections in Pregnancy**

(DHHS Updated Prevention and Treatment of Opportunistic Infections, *MMWR* 2009;58:RR11

Agent	Class*	Recommendation
Acyclovir	B	Treatment reserved for severe herpes or varicella; well-tolerated and no consequences with > 700 exposures
Albendazole	C	Teratogenic in rodents; reserve for severe microsporidiosis in 2nd and 3rd trimester
Amoxicillin	B	Standard indications
Amphotericin	B	Standard indications
Atovaquone	C	Standard indications; limited experience
Azithromycin	B	Standard indications
Caspofungin	C	Embryotoxic in rodents; no human experience
Cidofovir	C	Teratogenic in animals (black box warning); risk in women unknown
Ciprofloxacin	C	Arthropathy in beagle dogs; not recommended in pregnancy but > 400 cases of use with no arthropathy or birth defects
Clarithromycin	C	Teratogenic in animals; increased rate of abortions in women; azithromycin preferred for MAC
Clindamycin	B	Standard indications
Clotrimazole troche	C	No complications expected with oral or vaginal use
Dapsone	C	Limited experience; may increase risk of kernicterus
Doxycycline	D	Risk to infant teeth; avoid
Entecavir	C	Not teratogenic in rodents; no human data
Erythromycin	B	Standard indications
Ethambutol	C	Teratogenic at high doses in animal studies, appears safe in humans
Famciclovir	B	Limited data in humans; reserve for severe herpes
Fluconazole	C*	Bone defects in animals; reserve for severe and established fungal infections; Ampho B often preferred
Flycytosine	C	Bone defects in animals; use only after first trimester
Foscarnet	C	Teratogenic in animals and no data in humans; use for disseminated CMV

* Fluconazole is Class C for a single dose; Class D for multiple doses

TABLE 42: **Drugs for Opportunistic Infections in Pregnancy** *(cont.)*

Agent	Class*	Recommendation
Ganciclovir	C	Teratogenic in animals; limited but favorable experience in humans
Interferon	C	Delay treatment until after pregnancy
INH	C	Standard indications + pyridoxine
Itraconazole	C	Teratogenic in animals and concern for azoles in pregnancy; use for systemic mycosis; Ampho B often preferred
Mefloquine	C	May increase risk of stillbirth
Metronidazole	B	Extensive favorable experience in pregnant women; standard indications
Paromomycin	C	Not absorbed; fetal toxicity unlikely
Pentamidine	C	Embryocidal in animals; limited experience in women
Primaquine	C	Limited experience; theoretical risk of hemolytic anemia with G6PD deficiency
Posaconazole	C	Teratogenic in animals; risk in women unknown
Pyrazinamide	C	Not teratogenic in rodents; limited experience in humans
Pyrimethamine	C	Teratogenic in rodents; limited human experience suggests risk of birth defect; if used, add leucovorin
Ribavirin	X	Teratogenic in animals; not indicated in pregnancy
Rifabutin	B	Not teratogenic in animals
Rifampin	C	Teratogenic in animals; indicated for TB; vitamin K at birth
Sulfadiazine	C	Possible kernicterus if used near delivery
Telbivudine	B	Not teratogenic in rodents; limited data in humans
Valacyclovir	B	See acyclovir
Voriconazole	D	Teratogenic in rodents; Ampho B preferred

* **Classes:**
- **A** controlled studies show no risk
- **B** no evidence of risk in humans
- **C** risk not ruled out
- **D** positive evidence of risk
- **X** contraindicated in pregnancy

OPPORTUNISTIC INFECTIONS

Guidelines for the Prevention and Treatment of Opportunistic Infections in HIV-Infected Adults and Adolescents. *April 16, 2015.* Available at http://aidsinfo.nih.gov/contentfiles/lvguidelines/Adult_OI.pdf

TABLE 43: Guidelines for Prevention of Opportunistic Infections (2015 NIH/CDC/IDSA Guidelines)

Infection/Organism	Indication	First Choice
Strongly Recommended		
Pneumocystis jirovecii	• CD4 < 200/mm³ or • CD4% < 14%, thrush, hx of AIDS defining illness or FUO • CD4 <250/mm³ if q 3 months monitoring not possible	• TMP-SMX 1 DS/d* or • TMP-SMX 1 SS/d*
Myrobacterium tuberculosis	See Page 92 for latent or active TB and HIV Co-infection	
Toxoplasma gondii	+ anti-*Toxoplasma* IgG positive and CD4 < 100/mm³	• TMP-SMX 1 DS* qd
Mycobacterium avium complex	• CD4 < 50/mm³	• Azithromycin 1200 mg/wk or 600 mg po 2x/wk or • Clarithromycin 500 mg bid†
Varicella zoster	Post-exposure Chickenpox / shingles exposure and susceptible (no history of disease and varicella seronegative)	• VZIG 5 vials (6.25 mL) 125 IU/10 kg (max 625 IU) IM • < 96 h post exposure • Treatment IND 1-800-843-7477
	Pre-exposure No history of chickenpox, shingles, vaccine, or positive serology and CD4 count > 200/mm³	• Primary varicella vaccine (*Varivax*) (0.5 mL SQ) 2 doses 3 months apart

* SS= Single strength tablet, DS=Double strength tablet
† Dose adjusted for concurrent PI/NNRTI

Alternatives	Comments
ɔsone 100 mg/d or 50 mg bid or ɔsone 50 mg/d + pyrimethamine 50 /wk + leucovorin 25 mg/wk or 'osol pentamidine 300 mg by Respigard ebulizer once a month or vaquone 1500 mg +/- pyrimethamine mg + leucovorin 10 mg/d or P-SMX 1 DS* 3x/wk	• Discontinue prophylaxis if CD4 > 200/mm³ for > 3 mos • Restart prophylaxis if CD4 decreases to < 200/mm³ • Pyrimethamine regimens for toxoplasmosis prophylaxis • TMP-SMX 1DS/d provides toxoplasmosis prophylaxis • Avoid dapsone with G6PD deficiency
P-SMX 1 SS* qd or 1 DS 3x/week psone 50 mg/d + pyrimethamine 50 /wk + leucovorin 25 mg/wk psone 200 mg/wk + pyrimethamine 75 /wk + leucovorin 25 mg/wk ɔvaquone 1500 mg (± pyrimethamine 25 + leucovorin 10 mg)/d	• Discontinue prophylaxis if CD4 > 200/mm³ for ≥ 3 mos • Restart prophylaxis if CD4 decreases to < 100-200/mm³ • Repeat toxo serology if baseline serology negative and CD4 count subsequently declines to < 100/mm³
'abutin † 300 mg/d djust dose for concurrent ART)	• Discontinue prophylaxis if CD4 > 100/mm³ for ≥ 3 mos • Restart prophylaxis if CD4 decreases to < 50/mm³ • Rule out active MAC before giving monotherapy prophylaxis
:yclovir 800 mg 5x/d or valacyclovir 1 g ɔ8h x 5-7 days can be considered no data)	• Vaccinate household contacts to prevent transmission to susceptible HIV+ patient
	• Routine serology not recommended • If vaccine causes disease, treat with acyclovir

TABLE 44: **CDC/OI Guidelines for Vaccines in HIV-Infected Patients***

Infection/Organism	Indication	First Choice
Generally Recommended		
S. pneumoniae	• All patients with HIV regardless of CD4 count and no pneumococcal vaccine in 5 yrs • Consider if CD4 < 200/mm³	PCV 13 (*Prevnar 13*) 0.5 mL x 1, then PPSV23 (*Pneumovax*) 0.5 mL SC ≥ 8 weeks later, then in 5 years. ($152.01/dose) (MMWR 2012 61(40): 816) If prior PPSV23, PCV 13 ≥1 year la[t...] then a second dose PPSV23 ≥ 8 we[...] later, then in 5 years ($72.38/dose[)]
Hepatitis B	Susceptible (anti-HBc or anti-HBs negative) and HBsAg negative	HBV vaccine IM (*Engerix-B*) 20 mcg/mL or *Recombivax* 10 mcg/mL; Dose at 0, 1 and 6 mo ($52-61/dose)
Influenza	All patients annually regardless of CD4 count (seasonal)	Inactivated influenza vaccine 0.5 mL ($11-22/dose)
Hepatitis A	Susceptible (anti-HAV negative) and risk (IDU, MSM, travel) or chronic liver disease (HBV or HCV infection); persons receiving clotting factor concentrate.	• Hepatitis A vaccine series: 1.[...] x 2 at 0 and 6-12 mos (*Havrix*) ($64/dose) • Some delay until CD4 is > 200/mm³
Human papilloma virus (HPV)	Females and males, ages 11-12 yrs; 13-21 if unvaccinated. MSM, ages: up to age 26 Immunocompromised persons (HVI)-up to age 26	HPV vaccine bivalent (*Cervarix*) quadrivalent (*Gardasil*) 0.5 mL at 0, 2 & 6 mos ($147/dose)
Tetanus diphtheria and acellular pertussis (Tdap) Tetanus and diphtheria Toxoid (Td)	Female and males age 13-26	Single dose Tdap to all adults > 1[...] yrs who have not received Tdap ($40), then Td ($14) every 10 ye[...]
Varicella zoster	Age > 60 yrs and CD4 > 200/mm³ Contraindicated with CD4 < 200/mm³	*Zostavax* 0.65 mL SQ ($118) Varivax 0.5 mL SQ ($68)

* Recommendations are based on ACIP (CDC) 2015 (http://www.cdc.gov/vaccines/schedules/downloads/adult/adult-combined-schedule.pdf); Aberg J et al Primary Care Guideline for Management of Persons with HIV infection CID 2014; 58: e1; and Rubin LG et al 2013 IDSA Clinical Practice Guideline for Vaccination of the Immunocompromised Host CID 2013

Alternatives	Comments
	Consider reimmunization if CD4 increases to > 200/mm³ and initial immunization was given when CD4 < 200/mm³.
	Measure anti-HBs at one month after 3rd dose; if < 10 IU/mL: revaccinate w/ *Engerix*-B 40 mcg/mL or delay until CD4 count higher. Vaccination best when done w/ CD4 >350/mm³
:amivir 75 mg qd	*FluMist* (live virus vaccine) contraindicated regardless of CD4 count.
e	Determine antibody response 1 mo post-vaccination; if negative, revaccinate. HCV co-infected patient should be vaccinated. Give ≥ 2 weeks prior to travel. Consider Hep A + B (*Twinrix*) 1 ml in 3 doses (0, 1, and 6 mo) only for HAV and HBV non-immune.
	The quadrivalent vaccine HPV types 6, 11, 16, 18 is preferred in males. Some authorities recommend quadrivalent vaccine for MSM > 26 yrs in selected cases. 9 valent vaccine (Gardasil 9) adds protection against five additional HPV types—31, 33, 45, 52 and 58. Probably preferred, but recommendation not available.
	Tetanus prophylaxis in wound care: <3 prior doses or unknown vaccination, > 10 yrs post Td or severe injury >5 yrs
e	Zostavax vaccine can be considered in patients > 60 years old with CD4 count > 200/mm3 per HIVMA/IDSA primary care guidelines, but no data. Varicella vaccine (Varivax 2 doses separated 3 months apart) may be considered in VZV-seronegative adults with CD4 count > 200 /mm³ Susceptible patients (no Hx of varicella zoster and/or seronegative) should receive varicella immune globulin (*VariZig*) ASAP (within 10d of exposure to VZV).

Prices reported by private sector to CDC
http://www.cdc.gov/vaccines/programs/vfc/awardees/vaccine-management/price-list/

TABLE 45: **Treatment of Opportunistic Infections (NIH/CDC/IDSA)**

Infection/Organism	Treatment
Bartonella	**Bacillary angiomatosis, peliosis hepatitis, bacteremia, and osteomyelitis:** Erythromycin 500 mg qid po or IV x ≥ 3 mos or doxycycline 100 mg bid po or IV x ≥ 3 mos **Alternative:** Azithromycin 500 mg po/d x ≥ 3 mos or clarithromycin 500 mg bid po x ≥ 3 mos **CNS or severe infections:** Doxycycline 100 mg po or IV q12h +/- rifampin 300 mg po q12h or IV > 3 mos
Candida: **Thrush**	**Initial episode:** Fluconazole 100 mg po x 7-14 d or topical clotrimazole troches 10 mg po 5x/d or nystatin as susp 5 mL qid or as 1-2 flavored pastilles 4-5x/d x 7-14 d **Fluconazole refractory:** Itraconazole soln 200 mg/d po, posaconazole soln 400 mg bid po, amphotericin 0.3 mg/kg/d IV, anidulafungin 100 mg IV then 50 mg/d, casofungin 50 mg/d IV, micafungin 150 mg/d IV or ampho B susp 100 mg/mL 1 mL qid (mu be compounded by pharmacy)
Candida: **Esophagitis**	**Preferred:** Fluconazole 200 mg (up to 800 mg/d) po or IV x 14-21 **Fluconazole refractory:** Posaconazole soln 400 mg bid po x 28 d, ampho B 0.3-0.7 mg/kg/d IV or lipid ampho B 3-5 mg/kg/d, anidulafungin 100 mg IV then 50 mg/d IV, micafungin 150 mg/d IV, caspofungin 50 mg IV/d or voriconazole 200 mg bid po or IV
Candida: **Vaginitis**	**Preferred:** Fluconazole 150 mg po x 1 or topical azole x 3-7 d **Recurrent or complicated:** Fluconazole 150 mg po q72h x 2-3 or topical azole > 7 d
Cryptosporidium	**Preferred:** ART to achieve CD4 > 100/mm^3; antiotility agents and IV hydration **Alternative:** Nitazoxanide 0.5-1.0 gm po bid w/ food x 2 wks or paromomycin 500 mg po qid x 14-21 days.
Cryptococcal Meningitis	**Preferred:** Induction with liposomal amphotericin 3-4 mg/kg IV plus flucytosine 25 mg/kg qid po ≥ 2 wks then consolidation therapy with fluconazole 400 mg qd ≥ 8 wks, then maintenance therapy 200 mg/d **Alternative induction:** • Liposomal amphotericin 4-6 mg/kg/d IV or amphotericin B (alone) x4-6 wks • Ampho B 0.7 mg/kg/d IV + 5FC 25mg/kg qid x ≥ 2 wks • Fluconazole 1200 mg/d po or IV + flucytosine 100 mg/kg/d in 4 divided doses po x6 wks **Alternative-consolidation:** Itraconazole 200 mg po bid x 8 wks (less effective) **Alternative-maintenance:** Itraconazole 200 mg/d (less effective than fluconazole)

(continued)

Updated Opportunistic Infections Guidelines, 2015)

Comment
May need long-term suppression with doxycycline or macrolide if relapse until CD4> 200 cells/mm^3 May have severe Jarisch-Herxheilmer reaction in first 48 h Treat until CD4 > 200 cells for ≥ 6 months.
Alternative initial therapy: Itraconazole soln 200 mg/d po x 7-14 days. **Suppressive therapy:** Indicated for severe or frequent reoccurrences; fluconazole 100 mg/d or itraconazole soln 200 mg/d. Discontinue when CD4 > 200/mm^3.
Alternative initial therapy: Treat 14-21 d with itraconazole, voriconazole, posaconazole, caspofungin, micafungin, anidulafungin (prior designated doses) or ampho B 0.6 mg/kg/d IV **Suppressive therapy:** Indicated for severe or frequent reoccurrences fluconazole 100-200 mg po or posaconazole 400 mg bid po **Note:** Fluconazole refractory cases that responded to echinocandins may be transitioned to oral voriconazole or posaconazole prophylaxis
• **Alternative initial therapy:** Itraconazole soln 200 mg/d po x 3-7 d • **Maintenance:** Fluconazole 150 mg po q wk or daily topical azole
Antimotility agents: Loperamide or tincture of opium
• High opening pressure: LP to drain CSF until 50% OP. Repeat daily until OP < 200 mm Hg (this is critical). • Patients given 5FC should have blood levels measured to assure 2 h post dose level is 30-80 mg/mL (after 3-5 days). Adjust dose for renal failure. • Lipid amphotericin is preferred over ampho B due to equivalent efficacy and lower rate of nephrotoxicity and infusion reactions. • Addition of flucytosine to ampho B increases rate of CSF clearance of cryptococcus. • > 2 weeks induction recommended if PT has not clinically improved, with persistent ↑ ICP, and has positive CSF cultures at 2 weeks • After induction and consolidation phase, treat with fluconazole for at least a year and until CD4 count ≥ 100/mm^3 for >3 mos and VL <50 • Continue fluconazole maintenance lifelong or reinitiate fluconazole if CD4 <100/mm^3 • Delay initiation of ART until after 10 weeks of induction/consolidation antifungal. Earlier initiation may be considered in pts with severe immunosuppression (CD4 <50/mm^3)

(continued)

TABLE 45: Treatment of Opportunistic Infections *(cont.)*

Infection/Organism	Treatment
Cytomegalovirus: Retinitis	**Preferred for vision-threatening lesion:** Intravitreal ganciclovir (2r or foscarnet (2.4mg) x 1 to 4 doses over 7-10 days + valgancicloví 900 mg bid x 14-21 d, then 900 mg qd **Preferred for peripheral lesions:** Oral valganciclovir 900 mg bid p 14-21 d, then 900 mg qd **Alternatives:** • Ganciclovir 5 mg/kg bid IV x 14 d, then 5 mg/kg/d IV, or • Foscarnet 60 mg/kg q8h IV or 90 mg/kg q12h IV x 14 d, then 90-120 mg/kg IV qd, or • Cidofovir 5 mg/kg q7d IV x 2 doses, then 5 mg/kg q14d IV
Cytomegalovirus: Colitis, Esophagitis, Pneumonia	**Preferred:** Valganciclovir (oral), ganciclovir (IV), foscarnet (IV) per above doses for CMV retinitis x 21-42 d **Maintenance:** Role is unclear; consider after relapse
Cytomegalovirus: Neurologic Disease	**Preferred:** Ganciclovir + foscarnet as above for CMV retinitis **Maintenance:** IV foscarnet + po valganciclovir for life
Hepatitis B Virus (HBsAg+≥ 6 mos)	**Treatment for HIV:** At least 2 agents active versus both viruses (usually TDF/FTC) • 3TC/FTC-naive: TDF/FTC 300/200 mg/d (or TDF 300 mg/d + 3TC 3 mg/d) + additional agent for HIV • 3TC/FTC-experienced + detectable HBV DNA (assume 3TC/FTC/telbivudine resistance): Add TDF 300 mg qd + (3TC/FTC) or entecavir 1 mg/d (use only HIV viral load is undetectable) **Duration:** Both treated indefinitely **Treat HBV and not HIV:** • Usually treat both even with CD4 > 500/mm^3 • HBeAg- w/ HBV DNA < 2,000 IU/mL: Adefovir 10 mg/d po • HBeAg+ w/ HBV DNA > 20,000 IU/mL + ↑ ALT: Peg-interferon
Hepatitis C Virus	**See Table 52. Treatment of HCV**

Comment
stemic: Continue until inactive disease +CD4 > 100/mm^3 x 3-6 mos ohthalmology F/U required) q3 months. Reinitiate maintenance therapy if CD4 count 100 cells/mm^3. T critical component of treatment **mune recovery uveitis:** Periocular steroids or short course oral prednisone. raocular ganciclovir implant no longer available
aintenance: Consider after relapse or severe disease **IV pneumonia:** Indications are CMV by histology plus lack of response to other athogens **RT:** Critical component of treatment
RT is critical. ognosis pre-HAART was poor.
cations to treat HBV: Chronic HBV and • Treatment of HIV or • Standard recommendations for treating HBV: abnormal ALT + HBeAg + HBV DNA > 20,000 IU/mL or abnormal ALT + HBV DNA > 2,000 IU/mL with HBeAg neg **IV-coinfected and not receiving ART, treatment of HBV with the following agents can ult in HIV resistance:** • 3TC, FTC, TDF and entecavir **/HCV/HBV co-infection:** • Treat HIV/HBV first **Vhen changing HIV agents:** Maintain agents active against HBV **iscontinuation of anti-HBV agents:** May cause life-threatening flare - restart **elbivudine/FTC/3TC:** Assume cross-resistance

(continued)

TABLE 45: Treatment of Opportunistic Infections *(cont.)*

Infection/Organism	Treatment
Herpes Simplex: Mucocutaneous	**Preferred:** Valacyclovir 1 gm po bid, acyclovir 400 mg po tid, famciclovir 500 mg po bid x 5-10 days (orolabial) or x 5-14 days (genital) **Severe:** Acyclovir 5 mg/kg IV q8h, then oral agent for ≥ 21 d
Herpes Simplex: Keratitis	**Preferred:** Trifluridine 1% ophthalmic soln 1 drop q2h up to 9 drops/d ≤ 21 d
Herpes Simplex: Encephalitis	**Preferred:** Acyclovir 10 mg/kg q8h IV x 14-21 d
Microsporidia	**Preferred:** ART to get CD4 > 100/mm³ + rehydration Albendazole 400 mg po bid (intestinal and disseminated-not occula Treat until CD4 is > 200/mm³ x 6 mo. <u>Ocular:</u> Fumagillin (investigational in the US) topical-2 gtts q2h x 4 days, then 2 gtts qid until eye sx resolve and CD4 > 200/mm³ x 6 <u>Disseminated disease:</u> Itraconazole 400 mg po qd + albendazole 400 mg E. bleneusi **(20% of cases)**: Topical fumagillin 20 mg po tid or TNP- (not available in US) Treat until no signs and symptoms of microsporiodosis and CD4 > 200/mm³.
***Myobacterium avium* Complex**	**Preferred:** Clarithromycin 500 mg bid po + ethambutol 15 mg/kg OR azithromycin 500-600 mg qd po + ethambutol 15 mg/kg po qd **Adding a third/fourth drug should be considered w/ severe disea and CD4 < 50/mm³:** • rifabutin* 300 mg po qd • ciprofloxacin 500-750 mg bid po, • levofloxacin 500 mg qd po, or • moxifloxacin 400 mg qd po or • amikacin 10-15 mg/kg qd IV or • streptomycin 1 gm IM/d
Mycobacterium tuberculosis	See Tables 48-51
Pneumocystls jirovecii	**Preferred:** • TMP-SMX (15-20 mg/kg/d TMP and 75-100 mg SMX/kg/d) q6-8h IV; switch to po when clinically improved or • TMP-SMX 2 DS tid (TMP 5 mg/kg tid) x 21 d (for 70 Kg patient) **Alternative - severe disease:** • Pentamidine 4 mg/kg/d IV infused over > 60 min • Primaquine 30 mg po/d** + clindamycin 600-900 mg IV q6-8h or 450 mg po q6 x 21 days **Alternative - moderate or mild disease:** • Dapsone** 100 mg qd +TMP 5 mg/kg tid x 21 d; or • Primaquine** 30 mg base qd + clindamycin 450 mg po q6h x 21 or • Atovaquone 750 mg bid po with food x 21 d (less effective)

* Rifabutin reduces levels of clarithromycin by 50% (consider azithromycin if rifabutin is used). Rifabutin may need dose adjustment based on ART regimen.

Comment
yclovir-resistant HSV: Foscarnet 80-120 mg/kg/d IV in 2-3 daily doses **ternative:** Topical trifluridine, topical cidofovir, or topical imiquimod x 21-28 days **ronic suppressive treatment:** valacyclovir 500 mg bid, acyclovir 400 mg bid, or nciclovir 500 mg bid for severe HSV recurrences RVs may decrease severity of HSV episodes
tazoxanide has minimal efficacy against *E. bienensi* in pts with low CD4 count. **icrosporidia other than** *E. bieneusi*: Albendazole 400 mg bid po until D4 > 200/mm^3 **isseminated disease with** *Trachipleistophora* **or** *Brachiola*: Itraconazole 400 mg po qd albendazole 400 mg po bid. eat until no signs and symptoms of microsporidiosis and CD4 >200/mm^3 x 6 mos.
uration: Until MAC treatment ≥ 12 mos, asymptomatic and CD4 count > 100/mm^3 x mos. Reinitiate secondary est susceptibility to clarithromycin and azithromycin with clinical failure. SAIDs for symptoms attributed to IRIS; use 20-40 mg prednisone if IRIS symptoms persist se azithromycin to minimize CYP3A4 drug-drug interactions. dd 3rd or 4th drug (e.g RBT, moxifloxacin) should be considered in pt w/ severe disease nd CD4 count < 50/mm^3.
nitiate ART within 2 weeks of TB treatment in pts with CD4 < 50 cells/mm^3 and by 8-12 veeks for all others.
poxia (PaO_2 < 70 mm Hg or A-a O_2 gradient > 35 mm Hg): Start steroid ASAP. rednisone: 40 mg bid days 1-5, 40 mg qd days 6-10, then 20 mg qd days 11-21, or V methylprednisolone as 75% prednisone dose. **ilure to respond:** Jse alternative regimen but note that initial response is usually slow (e.g. > 5 d) condary Prophylaxis: TMP-SMX 1 DS once daily or TMP-SMX 1 SS once daily (preferred) Dapsone 100 mg/d OR dapsone 50 mg/d + pyrimethamine 50 mg/wk + leucovorin 25 ng/wk or Aerosol pentamidine 300 mg once per month by Respigard II nebulizer or Atovaquone 1500 mg +/- pyrimethamine 25 mg/d + leucovorin 10 mg/d

** Primaquine or dapsone: screening for G6PD recommended.

(continued)

TABLE 45: **Treatment of Opportunistic Infections** *(cont.)*

Infection/Organism	Treatment
Salmonella	**Preferred:** Ciprofloxacin 500-750 mg po (or 400 mg IV) q12h Alternative (if susceptible): • Moxifloxacin 400 mg po or IV q24h • Levofloxacin 750 mg po or IV q24 • TMP-SMX po or IV, *or* • Ceftriaxone 1 gm IV q24h, ***or*** Cefotaxime 1gm IV q8h
Toxoplasma gondii	**Preferred - acute** (treat for at least 6 wks): Pyrimethamine 200 mg x 1 po, then 50 mg (< 60 kg) or 75 mg (> kg) qd po + sulfadiazine 1 g (< 60 kg) or 1.5 g (> 60 kg) qid po + leucovorin 10-25 mg qd po x ≥ 6 wks. Continue longer if clinical or radiologic effect is extensive or response is delayed. **Alternative - acute:** • Pyrimethamine + leucovorin (as above) + one of the following: -Clindamycin 600 g q6h po or IV, ***or*** -Atovaquone 1500 mg bid po with food ***or*** -Azithromycin 900-1200 mg qd po • TMP-SMX 5 mg/kg bid IV or po, ***or*** • Atovaquone 1.5 g bid po with food ± sulfadiazine 1-1.5 g q6h po **Preferred - maintenance** (after ≥ 6 wk initial treatment): • Pyrimethamine 25-50 mg/d po + sulfadiazine 2-4 gm po/d in 2-4 doses + leucovorin 10-25 mg/d **Alternative - maintenance:** • Pyrimethamine 25-50 mg/d + leucovorin 10-25 mg po/d + clindamycin 600 mg q8h po • Atovaquone 750-1500 mg po q12h ± pyrimethamine 25 mg po qd + leucovorin 10 mg po/d ***or*** sulfadiazine 2-4 gm/d • Atovaquone 750-1500 mg po 12h + sulfadiazine 1-2 gm q12h • TMP/SMX 1DS po q12h

Comment
d gastroenteritis only and CD4 > 200/mm³: Treat 7-14 d; **CD4 count < 200/mm³:** Treat 2-6 wks **n recurrent gastroenteritis +/- bacteremia:** Treat until immune reconstitution (CD4 > /mm³ and VL < 50 c/mL)
djunctive dexamethasone given only if mass effect nticonvulsants if history of seizures. Check for drug-drug interactions between nticonvulsants and ARVs (see page 41). eat until free of signs and symptoms of toxo encephalitis and CD4 > 200/mm³ for > 6 onths. einitiate maintenance if CD4 count < 200/mm³.

TABLE 46: Immune Reconstitution Syndrome (IRIS)

Definition: MA French (CID 2004;18:1615)	
Must have major criteria A and B plus any two minor criteria	
Major Criteria	
A	Atypical presentation of an opportunistic infection or tumor in patients responding to ART • Localized disease with severe fever or pain • Exaggerated inflammatory response • Atypical inflammatory response such as necrosis, exaggerated granulomas, suppuration or perivascular lymphocytic local infiltrate • Progression or organ dysfunction or enlargement of preexisting lesion after definite improvement with pathogen specific treatment prior to ART plus exclusion of treatment toxicity and new alternative diagnosis
B	HIV VL decrease > 1-$\log_{10}$ c/mL
Minor Criteria	
• Increase CD4 count • Increase in immune response specific to the relevant pathogen such as skin test for TB • Spontaneous resolution of disease with ART and without disease-specific treatment	

Alternate Definition: Robertson, et al. (CID 2006 ;42 :1639)
• New or worsening symptoms of an infection or inflammatory condition after starting ART PLUS • Symptoms not explained by newly acquired infection, predicted course of previously diagnosed condition or adverse drug effects • HIV VL decrease > 1-$\log_{10}$ c/mL

OI	Clinical Features	Treatment/Comments
Common to all opportunistic infections	• Defined as a paradoxical worsening of a prior condition soon after starting ART • MAC and TB account for 30% of reported cases; less common with cryptococcal meningitis and CMV retinitis • Usually occurs at 1-8 wks post ART initiation • Baseline CD4 count is usually < 50/mm³ • Rapid reduction in HIV viral load • May occur while treating OI, at time of OI clinical stability or as newly detected OI	• Usual treatment is to continue ART, antimicrobial therapy agents for the OI, and give NSAIDs and/or steroids if severe IRIS • ACTG A5164 compared early ART (<14 days from OI dx) vs delayed (42-84 days). Early ART improved survival. • IRIS reportedly rare with: histoplasmosis, aspergillosis, bartonellosis, cryptosporidiosis, and Candida sp.

TABLE 47: Immune Reconstitution Syndrome

(Adapted from *Clin Infect Dis* 2004;38:1159 and 2016 DHHS Opportunistic Infection Guidelines)

Agent	Clinical Features	Treatment/Comments
***M. avium* complex**	Focal adenitis with systemic IRIS simulating TB IRIS. Expression highly variable with adenitis, Other expressions-pulmonary infiltrates, liver granuloma, mediastinitis, osteomyelitis, cerebritis	• ART, antibiotics, ± NSAIDs or high dose steroids • Common cause of IRIS-10% of cases
M. tuberculosis	Hectic fevers, worsening adenopathy, new and worsening pulmonary infiltrates. Severe IRIS: enlarging cerebral tuberculomas, meningitis, pericardial effusions, extensive pulmonary lesions, splenomegaly. Incidence is 16% and fatality rate 3.2%. Other expression include ARDS, adenitis, hepatitis, renal failure, epididymitis	• ART, anti-TB meds, NSAIDS ± high dose steroids • ART is favored but rate of IRIS is 6-23%
Cryptococcus	Worsening clinical meningitis despite microbiological response. Other expressions-palsy, hearing loss, abscess, mediastinitis, adenitis, fever, pneumonia, pleural effusion.	• Continue ART and antifungal therapy and reduce intracranial pressure if indicated. Use of short course steroid is arbitrary. • ACTG A5164 favored early earlier ART, but some studies show worse outcome.
P. jirovecii	Pneumonia	ART, anti-PCP meds, steroids
PML (JC virus)	IRIS possible in first wks or months of ART with CNS lesions showing contrast enhancement, edema and mass effect	High dose steroids with taper over 1-6 weeks. Contrast MRI at 2-6 weeks helpful.
HSV	Chronic erosive ulcers, encephalitis	ART, antivirals, steroids
Varicella zoster	Zoster flare	ART, antivirals
CMV	Retinitis-inflammation in anterior chamber or vitreous; can lead to vision loss. Cytoid macular edema, uveitis	ART, steroids + anti-CMV agents. Periocular, intravitreal, or systemic steroid administration all reported effective
KS	New onset KS or exacerbation of previously stable disease including tracheal mucosal edema, obstruction	ART +/- steroids
Hepatitis B	Hepatitis fare with elevated ALT and AST	ART active against HBV. Must distinguish ART-agent hepatotoxicity (or other causes), but need to discontinue ART is rare. Liver biopsy may show eosinophils (drug toxicity) or portal inflammation (viral hepatitis)
HPV	Inflamed warts	Steroids, surgery
HSV	Atypical mucocutaneous lesions refractory to HSV therapy (rare)	ART, antiviral
Toxoplasma	Encephalitis	ART, Steroids

TREATMENT OF TUBERCULOSIS

(American Thoracic Society / Centers for Disease Control and Prevention / Infectious Diseases Society of America: Treatment of Tuberculosis *Am J Respir Crit Care Med* 2003;167(4):603; http://www.cdc.gov/tb/topic/treatment, and NIH/CDC/IDSA Updated Opportunistic Infections Guidelines, 2014)

TABLE 48: Latent TB and HIV Co-Infection

Candidates for tuberculosis skin test (TST) or interferon gamma release assay (IGRA):

- Screen with TST or IGRA. IGRA is more sensitive, has less cross-reactivity with other mycobacteria
- IGRA is preferred in patients with recent BCG
- All HIV-infected patients without prior positive test upon entry into HIV care
- Repeat testing annually for HIV-infected patients at risk of acquiring TB who have no prior positive tests
- All HIV-infected patients with prior negative skin test who are discovered to be contacts of pulmonary cases

Indications for treatment of latent tuberculosis infection

- Positive PPD (≥ 5 mm induration) or positive IGRA plus no prior completed prophylaxis or treatment for TB disease
- Recent contact with TB case. Recent contacts who are initially TST negative should have TST repeated 12 wks after last exposure to TB case. Those placed on prophylaxis should be discontinued if PPD negative at 12 wks.
- History of inadequately treated TB that healed
- Rule out active TB based on symptoms, chest x-ray, sputum AFB and cultures or *Xpert* molecular test

Treatment of latent tuberculosis

- **Preferred Regimens:**
  1) INH 300 mg + pyridoxine 25 mg qd for 9 mos (270 doses in 12 mos); or
  2) INH 900 mg 2x/wk + pyridoxine 25 mg/d by directly observed therapy for 9 mos (76 doses in 12 mos)
- **Alternative Regimens:**
  - Rifampin 10 mg/kg (600 mg max) x 4 mos or
  - Rifabutin with dose adjustment based on ARV regimen x 4 mos
  - Rifapentine + INH x 3 months DOT. Not recommended in HIV-infected patients on interacting ARVs (e.g PI/r, NNRTIs, EVG, DTG)
- **MDR-TB Exposure:** Expert consultation is recommended for persons who are likely to be infected with INH- and RIF- (multidrug) resistant-TB and at high risk of reactivation

Monitoring therapy

- Contact monthly to review symptoms suggesting hepatitis
- LFTs (ALT and bilirubin) at baseline, 1 mo, 3 mos, and with symptoms of hepatitis. D/C INH if asymptomatic and ALT increases to ≥ 5x ULN or if symptomatic and ALT increases to ≥ 3x ULN

TABLE 49: Treatment of Drug-Susceptible Active Tuberculosis†

Phase 1 (8 wks)	Phase 2 (4-7 mos)*: Regimen, Doses, MInimal Duration
INH, RIF, PZA, EMB 8 wks • 7 d/wk for 8 wks (56 doses); or • 5 d/wk for 8 wks (40 doses)	• INH/RIF 7 d/wk for 18 wks (126 doses); or • INH/RIF 5 d/wk for 18 wks (90 doses); or • INH/RIF 2 x/wk for 18 wks (36 doses)
INH, RIF, PZA, EMB 2 wks/6 wks • 7d/wk, for 2 wks (14 doses), then • 2 x/wk for 6 wks (12 doses)	• INH/RIF 2x/wk for 18 wks (36 doses)
INH, RIF, PZA, EMB 8 wks • 3 x/wk for 8 wks (24 doses)	• INH/RIF 3x/wk for 18 wks (54 doses)
INH, RIF, EMB 8 wks • 7 d/wk for 8 wks (56 doses); or • 5 d/wk for 8 wks (40 doses)	• INH/RIF 7 d/wk for 31 wks (217 doses); or • INH/RIF 5 d/wk for 31 wks (155 doses); or • INH/RIF 2 x/wk for 31 wks (62 doses)

INH = Isoniazid, **RIF** = Rifampin, **PZA** = Pyrazinamide, **EMB** = Ethambutol

* Patients with cavitation at baseline or positive cultures at 2 mos should receive 31 wks continuation phase for total of 9 mos

† Directly observed therapy (DOT) recommended for all patients with HIV-related active TB. Note that total doses is considered more important than total duration

TABLE 50: Doses of Antituberculosis Drugs – First Line Drugs

Drug	5-7 daily per wk	2 x/wk	3 x/wk
INH*	5 mg/kg (300)*†	15 mg/kg (900)*†	15 mg/kg (900)*†
RIF*	10 mg/kg (600)*	10 mg/kg (600)*	10 mg/kg (600)*
PZA (wt) 40-55 kg 56-74 kg 76-90 kg	 1.0 gm 1.5 gm 2.0 gm	 2.0 gm 3.0 gm 4.0 gm	 1.5 gm 2.5 gm 3.0 gm
EMB (wt) 40-55 kg 56-74 kg 76-90 kg > 90 kg	 800 mg 1200 mg 1600 mg 1600 mg	 2000 mg 2800 mg 4000 mg 4000 mg	 1200 mg 2000 mg 2400 mg 2400 mg

* Usual dose in mg in parentheses.

† INH should be given with pyridoxine. Dose at 25 mg on each day INH is given.

TABLE 51: **Special Considerations for TB Treatment with HIV Co-Infection**

Special issues for TB/HIV co-infection
All patients with HIV should be evaluated for TB and all TB patients should be evaluated for HIV
Risk of active TB increases with decline in CD4 count, but the increase risk is noted early in HIV disease with the CD4 count is > 500/mm³
Always treat TB first and do not start concurrent therapy due to pill burden and overlapping toxicity (rash, hepatitis, GI intolerance)
-Timing of ART base of CD4 and disease severity (see below).
IRIS is common and is most frequent with a baseline CD4 < 100/mm³ and with treatment initiated in first 2 mos. Clinical features include high fevers, deceasing respiratory function, adenopathy, CNS lesions, and pleural effusions.
-Treatment is symptomatic with non-steroids is preferred, but steroid for severe IRIS reactions.
Steroids:Adjunctive steroids improve survival with HIV-associated TB pericarditis or TB meningitis
Suggested steroid regimen with rifampin based regimen-Prednisone 1.5 mg/kg/d x 2 weeks, then 0.75 mg/kg/d x 2 weeks
Suggested steroid regimen with rifabutin based regimen-Prednisone 1.0 mg/kg/d x 2 weeks, then 0.5 mg/kg/d x 2 weeks
Drug-drug Interactions between rifampin and rifapentine and ART:
-EFV-based ART can be given using standard regimens;
-PI-based ART requires use of rifabutin in place of rifampin with modified doses of the PI (see page 36)
-TAF should be avoided with all rifamycin including rifabutin
-EVG/COBI/TDF/FTC-avoid with rifampin
-DTG 50 mg BID or RAL 800 mg BID plus 2NRTIs can be used with rifampin

Duration of treatment
• **Acute phase**: 2 mos-INH/(RIF or RBT)/EMB/PZA with discontinuation of EMB if strain is pan-sensitive
• **Continuation phase**: INH/(RIF or RBT) tiw or (if CD4 > 100/mm³) biw x 4-10 mos
• **Total duration**
• *Pulmonary TB without cavity and neg sputum at 2 mo: 6 mo*
• *Pulmonary TB + cavity or positive sputum at 2 mo: 9 mo*
• *Extrapulmonary TB with CNS, bone, or joint involvement: 9-12 mos*
• *Extrapulmonary TB at other sites: 6-9 mos*

Timing of starting ART with TB/HIV (2012 DHHS Guidelines)
• **CD4 < 50**: Start ART within 2 weeks of starting TB treatment
• **CD4 ≥ 50 plus severe HIV disease**: Start ART within 2-4 wks
• **CD4 > 50 (other)**: ART can be delayed 2-4 wks but should be started by wk 8-12 of TB treatment

TABLE 52: **Treatment of Hepatitis C:**

(Amer Assoc for Study of Liver Diseases (AALSD) and Infectious Disease Society of America (IDSA)
(http://www.hcvguidelines.org)

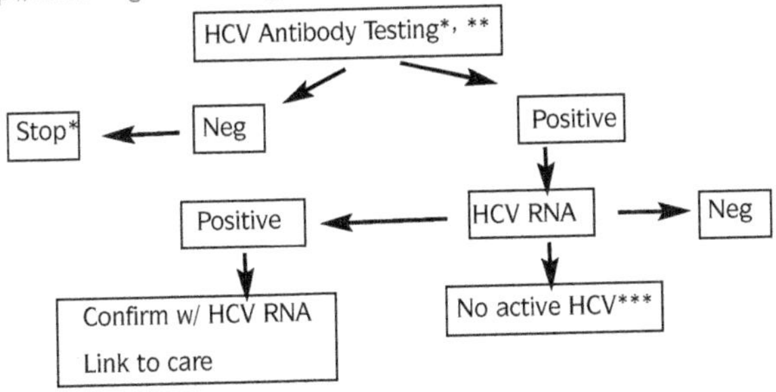

*<u>Risk for HCV:</u> Birth cohort: Born between 1945-1965 or other risk factor: IDU, hemodialysis, healthcare risk injury from HCV source, transfusion, organ transplant before 1992, or clotting factor concentrates before 1987, incarceration, <u>HIV infection</u>, unexplained liver disease, solid organ donor
**Anual testing for IDUs, HIV-infected MSM with unprotected sex
*** Retest Ab or HCV RNA recommended if risk within the past 6 months.

Active HCV infection
1) Patient education concerning transmission risks; 2) patient should avoid ETOH; 3) Evaluate for concurrent hepatic risks-HBV and HIV serology; 4) Vaccinate for HAV and HBV if not immune
Evaluation
Evaluate for fibrosis: Liver biopsy, *Fibroscan*, or non-invasive biomarkers Evaluation by a practitioner who can provide comprehensive care including antiviral HCV therapy
Goal of Treatment
Sustained viral response, i.e cure
Candidates for Treatment
All HCV infected patients can benefit from treatment <u>Highest Priorities for HCV treatment:</u> 1) Advanced fibrosis (metavir F3) or compensated cirrhosis [metavir F4]) 2) Organ transplant 3) Type 2 or 3 essential mixed cryoglobulinemia with end organ involvement (vasculitis) 4) Proteinuria, nephrosis, or membranoproliferative glomerulonephritis <u>High Priorities for HCV treatment</u> due to high risk of complications: HIV-coinfection, metavir F2, HBV co-infection, additional source of liver disease (eg NASH, debilitating fatigue, type2 insulin resistant diabetes, porphyria cutanea tarda <u>Priority based on elevated risk of HCV transmission:</u> High risk MSM, active IDU, incarcerated persons, long term hemodialysis, women with child-bearing potential desiring pregnancy, healthcare workers who perform invasive procedures.

TABLE 52: **Treatment of Hepatitis C:**

(Amer Assoc for Study of Liver Diseases (AALSD) and Infectious Disease Society of Ameri
(IDSA) (http://www.hcvguidelines.org accessed 08/14/2015)

Treatment naive w/ genotype 1a

1) Daily fixed-dose combination of elbasvir (50 mg)/grazoprevir (100 mg) x 12 weeks in patients without cirrhosis or compensated cirrhosis. Do not use if baseline high fold-change NS5A RAVs (G1a polymorphisms at amino acid positions 28A/G/T, 30D/E/H/G/K/L/R, 31F/M/V, or 93C/H/N/S) for elbasvir are detected.

2) Daily fixed-dose combination of ledipasvir (90 mg) + sofosbuvir (400 mg) x12 weeks in pts without cirrhosis or compensate cirrhosis

3) Daily fixed-dose combination of paritaprevir (150 mg)/ritonavir (100 mg)/ombitasvir (25 mg) plus bid dasabuvir (250 mg) and weight-based RBV** x 12 wks (no cirrhosis) or x24 wks (alternative in pts with compensated cirrhosis)

4) Daily sofosbuvir (400 mg) plus simeprevir (150 mg) x 12 weeks (no cirrhosis) or 24 weeks +/- weight-based RBV** (alternative in pts with compensated cirrhosis)

5) Daily daclatasvir* (60 mg) and sofosbuvir (400 mg) x 12 weeks (no cirrhosis) or x 24 weeks +/- RBV** (alternative in pts with compensated cirrhosis)

Treatment naive w/ genotype 1b

1) Daily fixed-dose combination of elbasvir (50 mg)/grazoprevir (100 mg) x 12 weeks in patients without cirrhosis or compensated cirrhosis.

2) Daily fixed-dose combination of ledipasvir (90 mg) + sofosbuvir (400 mg) x12 weeks (in pts without cirrhosis or compensate cirrhosis)

3) Daily fixed-dose combination of paritaprevir (150 mg)/ritonavir (100 mg)/ombitasvir (25 mg) plus bid dasabuvir (250 mg) x 12 weeks. (in pts without cirrhosis or compensate cirrhosis)

4) Daily sofosbuvir (400 mg) plus simeprevir (150 mg) x 12 weeks (no cirrhosis) or 24 weeks +/- weight-based RBV** (alternative in pts with compensated cirrhosis)

5) Daily daclatasvir* (60 mg) and sofosbuvir (400 mg) x 12 weeks (no cirrhosis) or x 24 weeks +/- RBV** (alternative in pts with compensated cirrhosis)

Treatment naive w/ genotype 2

Daily sofosbuvir (400mg) plus weight-based RBV** x 12 weeks (no cirrhosis) OR sofosbuvir (400mg) daily plus daclatasvir* (60mg) daily x 12 wks (no cirrhosis) in patients with contraindications to RBV. With compensated cirrhosis, extend treatment duration to 16-24 weeks.

Treatment naive w/ genotype 3

Daily daclatasvir* (60 mg) and sofosbuvir (400 mg) x 12 weeks (no cirrhosis) or x 24 weeks +/- RBV** (compensated cirrhosis)

Daily sofosbuvir (400 mg) plus weight-based RBV** and weekly PEG-IFN x 12 wks (no cirrhosis)

Extend treatment duration to 24 wks in pts with compensated cirrhosis

Contraindications to Peg-IFN or daclatasvir: sofosbuvir (400mg) once-daily plus weight based RBV** can be used as an alternative regimen in pts without cirrhosis or compensate cirrhosis.

**Weight based ribavirin (RBV) dosing: <75kg=1000 mg/d in two divided doses; >75kg=1200 mg/d in two divided doses.

*Daclastavir dose may need to be adjusted based on co-administered CYP3A4 inhibitors or inducers (e.g with ATV/r: use daclastavir 30mg/d; with EFV, NVP, ETR: use daclastavir 90mg/d)

See Table 17 (page 49) for anti-HCV and ARV drug-drug interactions

Treatment naive w/ genotype 4 1) Daily fixed-dose combination of paritaprevir (150 mg)/ritonavir (100 mg)/ombitasvir (25 mg) and weight-based RBV** x 12 wks (in pts without cirrhosis or compensate cirrhosis) 2) Daily fixed-dose combination of ledipasvir (90 mg)+ sofosbuvir (400 mg) x 12 wks (in pts without cirrhosis or compensated cirrhosis). 3) Daily fixed-dose combination of elbasvir (50 mg)/grazoprevir I 00 mg) x 12 weeks in patients without cirrhosis or compensated cirrhosis. Alternative: 1) Daily sofosbuvir (400 mg) and weight-based RBV** plus weekly PEG-IFN x 12 weeks
Treatment naive w/ genotype 5 Daily fixed-dose combination of ledipasvir (90 mg) plus sofosbuvir (400 mg) x 12 wks. (in pts without cirrhosis or compensate cirrhosis) Alternative: Daily sofosbuvir (400 mg) plus weight-based RBV** plus weekly PEG-IFNx 12 wks (in pts without cirrhosis or compensate cirrhosis) **Treatment naive w/ genotype 6** Daily fixed-dose combination of ledipasvir (90 mg) plus sofosbuvir (400 mg) x 12 wks (in pts without cirrhosis or compensate cirrhosis) Alternative: Daily sofosbuvir (400 mg) plus weight-based RBV** plus weekly PEG-IFNx 12 wks (in pts without cirrhosis or compensate cirrhosis)
HCV Treatment experienced: see www.hcvguidelines.org

**Weight based ribavirin (RBV) dosing: <75kg=1000 mg/d in two divided doses; >75kg=1200 mg/d in two divided doses.
*Daclastavir dose may need to be adjusted based on co-administered CYP3A4 inhibitors or inducers (e.g with ATV/r: use daclastavir 30mg/d; with EFV, NVP, ETR: use daclastavir 90mg/d)
See Table 17 (page 49) for anti-HCV an ARV drug-drug interactions

TABLE 53: Sexually Transmitted Disease*

(CDC 2015 STD guidelines http://www.cdc.gov/std/tg2015/)

Condition	Clinical Presentation/ Screening	Diagnosis
Urethritis/ Cervicitis	• Sx: Male-dysuria; urethral discharge; Female-cervical discharge+/- friable cervix • Many cases are asymptomatic • Ethiolgic agents: GC and non-gonococcal (*C. trachomatis, M genitalium*, Trichomonas and others) • Review of hx at follow-up visits, including contacts	*N. gonorrhoeae* + *C. Trachomatis*: test first voided urine. Alternative: 1st voided urine for Gr methylene blue, or gentian violet s detect gonococci (intracellular diplo Inflammation (>2 WBC/oil immersi field) with neg GC stain is presump *trachomatis*.
Gonorrhea	• Dx: NAAT test-1st void urine and vaginal swabs (NAAT tests appropriate for rectal and pharyngeal swabs, though not FDA approved) • Sequela in females: PID, ectopic pregnancy and infertility. • Most common presentation: urethritis or cervicitis • Extra-genital sites of GC infection: oropharyngeal, rectal, conjunctival, and disseminated (DGI) • Review of Hx at follow-up visits, including contact with known other cases • Many infections are asymptomatic in men and women: consider urinary NAAT for GC & CT in sexually active men and women, including contacts with established cases. • Pharyngeal and anal testing in at risk patients	Gram stain or methylene blue and/ culture (or other specific test) of ur or cervical swabs. Urine NAAT tests valid for urethral infections, are mo sensitive and usually more acceptal patients. Limitation is lack of antibi sensitivities. Alternative agent: *M. genitalium*
Chlamydia	• Patient self-report Sx • Review of Hx at follow-up visits, including contacts • Most infections are asymptomatic • Consider as routine cervical test for sexually active women < 25 yrs. Consider routine NAAT urine test for GC & CT in sexually active women > 25 yrs and men • Consider repeat test annually, or more often with high risk	Culture is infrequently available. Alternatives are OFA, EIA, and NAAT urethral and cervical specimens. Urine NAAT tests are sensitive and c preferred
Syphilis	• Patient self-report Sx • Contact with case • Screen at initial visit • Repeat screen annually	• Non-treponemal test (VDRL or RPR) plu treponemal test (FTA-ABS, TP-PA or EIA) • Non-treponemal test (RPR, VDRL) titers disease activity including response to treatment • Darkfield exam or OFA of lesion mater

† Screening interval depends upon community prevalence, outcome of previous tests, and risk

‡ Tetracycline, fluoroquinolones contraindicated in pregnancy

Treatment
mptive treatment of GC/CT for patients at risk (< 25 yrs, new sex partner, sex partner concurrent partners, or sex partner w/ STDs) rsistent and recurrent non-GC urethritis, consider *Mycoplasma genitallium* that is cated in 30% of non-GC cases. If initially treated with doxycycline: give azithromycin 1gm ially treated with azithromycin: give moxifloxacin 400 mg once daily x 7days rosexual men in a high *T. vaginalis* prevalence area: metronidazole 2g x1 or tinidazole 2 1
ral, endocervical, rectal, pharyngeal: Ceftriaxone 250 mg IM x 1 plus azithromycin 1gm po x 1 1 if *C. trachomatis* is ruled out) 2015 changes in treatment recs are based on resistance reported to cefixime and increasing to doxycycline. Treatment failure to cephalosporin should prompt culture and sensitivity ıg. **native to azithromycin:** Doxycycline 100 mg bid x 7 days. **Alternative to ceftriaxone:** me 400mg x 1 **alosporin allergy:** gemifloxacin 320 mg x1 PLUS azithromycin 2 gm (plus test-of-cure at 1) OR gentamicin 240 mg IM x 1 PLUS azithromycin 2gm njunctivitis: ceftriaxone 1gm IM plus azithromycin 1gm x1 x partners for past 60 days: Refer for evaluation and treatment st of cure testing recommended for pharyngeal GC
eminated GC: x: Culture or NAAT testing from multiple sites plus sensitivity testing. thritis-Dermatitis: Ceftriaxone1 gm/d IM or IV until improved for 24-48 h plus azithromycin po x 1, then ≥ 1 wk treatment with oral agents based on sensitivity tests: cefixime 400 mg qd profloxacin 500 mg bid or ofloxacin 400 mg bid or levofloxacin 500 mg qd. High rates of oquinolone resistance reported nationally; check local resistance pattern
nromycin** 1 gm po x 1 or ycycline‡** 100 mg po bid x 7 d **gnancy:** Azithromycin 1gm po x 1 **rnative:** Amoxicillin 500 mg tid x 7 d or erythromycin regimen (above doses) ailure with doxycycline: Azithromycin 1 gm x 1. Failure with azithromycin: moxifloxacin) mg/d x 7 d onsider pharyngeal and anal testing in at risk patients

Table 54: Management of Syphillis Co-Infection: Summary

(continued)

TABLE 53: **Sexually Transmitted Disease*** *(cont.)*

(CDC 2015 STD guidelines http://www.cdc.gov/std/tg2015/)

Condition	Identification / Screening	Diagnosis
Herpes simplex	• Recurrent genital ulcers • Most common cause of genital ulcer disease in the US and the world • Many infections are asymptomatic with viral shedding and transmission	• Patients with lesions suspectec herpes should be evaluated. • PCR is preferred test; culture, test and IAFA are less sensitive • Serology for HSV-2 most sensit test for HSV-2 infection, but nc Dx of herpes outbreak
Trichomonas	Malodorous yellow-green vaginal discharge	Wet mount or culture; NAAT is hi sensitive and detects 3-5 fold mc cases compared to wet-mount microscopy
Bacterial Vaginosis	"Fishy smelling" vaginal discharge	3 of the following: • Clue cells (vaginal epithelial cel with adherent coccobacillus) • pH vaginal fluid > 4.5 • Fishy odor with 10% KOH • Thin white discharge on vaginal
Pelvic inflammatory disease	Diverse symptoms reflecting inflammation of the upper female genital tract with endometritis and salpingitis. Suspect with sexually active female with unexplained pelvic or lower abdominal pain. Physical exam shows cervical motion, uterine and/or adnexal tenderness.	• Oral temp >101° F • Mucopurulent cervical discharge • Vaginal fluid with abundant WB • Increased ESR, CRP • Diagnosis of GC or CT

* CDC STD treatment guidelines updated by authors to reflect latest research data

Treatment			
	Acyclovir	Famciclovir	Valacyclovir
nd no HIV			
Episode	400 mg tid x 7-10 d	250 mg tid x 7-10 d	1 gm bid x 7-10 d
dic	400 mg tid x 5 d or 800 mg bid x 5 d or 800 mg tid x 2 d	125 mg bid x 5 d or 1000 mg bid x 1 d	500 mg bid x 3 d or 1 gm qd x 5 d
ession	400-800 mg tid	250 mg bid	500 mg or 1gm qd
nd HIV			
dic	400 mg bid or tid x 5-10 d	500 mg bid x 7-10 d	1 gm bid x 5-10 d
ession	400-800 mg bid or tid	500 mg bid	500 mg bid

nidazole 2 gm 1X OR metronidazole 500 mg bid x 7 d
regimen fails, metronidazole or tinidazole 2g once-daily x 7 days. Test susceptibility.

onidazole 500 mg bid x 7 d OR metronidazole gel 0.75% 5g intravaginal qd x 5 d OR
amycin 2% cream 5g intravaginally qhs x 7 d
ative: Tinidazole 2g po qd x 2 d; tinidazole 1g po qd x 5 d; clindamycin 300 mg bid x 7
ndamycin ovules 100 mg intravaginally qhs x 3 d.

muscular/Oral regimen
axone 250 mg IM x 1 plus doxycycline 100 mg bid x 14 d +/- metronidazole 500 mg po
d
xitin 2 gm x 1 plus probenicid 1 gm po x 1 plus doxycycline 100 mg bid x 14 d +/-
onidazole 500 mg po x 14 d
r 3rd generation cephalosporin plus doxycycline 100 mg bid x 14 d +/- metronidazole 500
o x 14 d

nteral: Cefoxitin 2 gm IV q6h OR cefotetan 2gm IV q12h
US doxycycline 100 mg po or IV q12h until improved,
EN doxycycline 100 mg bid po to complete 14 d
nteral alternative: Ampicillin/sulbactam 3gm IV q6h
US doxycycline IV or PO 100 mg q12h to complete 14 d course

TABLE 54: Management of Syphilis Co-Infection: Summary*

Form	Treatment	LP†
Primary and secondary syphilis	• **Initial:** Benzathine penicillin G 2.4 mil units IM x 1 • **Penicillin allergy:** doxycycline 100 mg po bid x 14 d or ceftriaxone 1 gm qd IV or IM x 8-10 d or azithromycin 2 gm po x 1 • **Re-treatment:** Benzathine penicillin G 2.4 mil units IM x 3 (weekly)	• Neuro SX • Titer increases 4 • SX persist or rec
Early latent (< 1 year)	• **Initial:** Benzathine penicillin G 2.4 mil units IM x 1 • **Penicillin allergy:** doxycycline 100 mg po bid x 14 d or ceftriaxone 1 gm qd IV or IM x 8-10 d or azithromycin 2 gm po x 1 • **Re-treatment:** Benzathine penicillin G 2.4 mil units IM x 3 (weekly)	• Neuro SX • SX persist or rec
Late latent (> 1 year or unknown duration)	• Benzathine penicillin G 2.4 mil units IM weekly for 3 weeks • **Penicillin allergy:** doxycycline 100 mg po bid x 28 days‡	• All HIV-infected patients
Late syphilis (tertiary, not neurosyphilis)	• Benzathine penicillin G 2.4 mil units IM weekly for 3 weeks • **Penicillin allergy:** doxycycline 100 mg po bid x 28 days‡	• All patients
Neurosyphilis ** (or ocular syphilis)	• Aq penicillin G, 18-24 mil units/d x 10-14 d administered as 3-4 million units IV q4h • Alternative: Procaine penicillin 2.4 million units IM qd + probenecid 500 mg po qid x 10-14 d • **Penicillin allergy:** ceftriaxone 2 gm qd IV or IM x 10-14 d (risk of cross-reaction is low but not zero. Skin testing to confirm allergy and/or PCN desensitization with consultant expertise, then treat with penicillin (preferred).	• Required

* CDC 2015 STD treatment guidelines and 2015 OI guidelines

† Some experts recommend CSF examinations of all syphilis-H IV co-infected patients before treatment, regardless of stage, and modification of treatment accordingly. Consultation with an expert may be appropriate.

‡ Alteratives to penicillin have not been sufficiently evaluated in HIV infected persons and cannot be considered first-line therapy. If required, there needs to be close clinical monitoring. If adherence cannot be assured, desensitization and treatment with penicillin is recommended.

**CSF VDRL is very specific bu not very sensitive. It is the only approved CSF syphilis test. Consider CNS syphilis if other conditions ruled out and CSF WBC >20. Note that CSF FTA-abs is not specific but may help rule out neurosyphilis (Harding AS, Sex Trans Dis 2012; 39: 291)

-up VDRL/RPR	Expectation VDRL/RPR	Indications to Re-treat
, 6, 9, 12, ıd 24 mos	4-fold decrease at 6-12 mos	• Titer increases four-fold • Titer fails to decrease four-fold at 6-12 mos • Symptoms persist or recur
6, 12, 18, nd 24 mos	4-fold decrease at 12-24 mos	• Titer increases four-fold • Titer of > 1:32 fails to decrease four-fold at 12-24 mos • Develops signs or sx of syphilis
, 6, 12, 18, nd 24 mos	4-fold decrease at 6-12 mos (lower initial titers may remain unchanged)	• Titer fails to decrease four-fold at 12-24 mos • Increase titer by four-fold at any time after 3 mos
and 12 mos	• As above • Granulomatous lesions should heal	• As above • Documentation of *T. pallidum* or other histologic features of late syphilis
:very 6 mos :il CSF normal	CSF WBC decrease at 6 mos and CSF normal at 24 mos	• CSF WBC fails to decrease at 6 mos or CSF VDRL is still positive • Persisting signs and symptoms

TABLE 55: **Occupational Post·Exposure Prophylaxis (PEP)**

(MMWR 2015; 63: 1245 and Kuhar DT Infect Control Hosp Epidemiol 2013; 34 (9): 875)

Exposure

Percutaneous injury with sharp object or exposure to mucous membranes or nonintact skin (skin that is abraded, chapped or with dermatitis)

Risk

- US data from occupational HIV transmissions for 1985 to 2013: 58 confirmed and 150 possible cases. There was only one confirmed case from 2000-2012 (Joyce MP MMWR 2015; 63: 1245)
- Prospective studies of transmission risk in the pre-HAART era showed 1) 20/6135 (0.33%) following percutaneous exposure; 2) 1/1143 (0.09%) following mucous membrane exposure; and 3) 0/2712 intact skin exposures (Henderson DK. Ann Intern Med 1990; 113: 740). More recent CDC guidance still quote a risk of 0.3% for occupationally-acquired HIV with a needlestick injury from an HIV infected source despite more recent low number of reported events with only one confirmed case in U.S. (Henderson DK. JAMA 2012; 307:75)

Management

Exposed site: Immediate cleansing of exposed site-1) skin: soap and water; 2) puncture wounds: alcohol-based hand wipes; 3) mucosal surface: flush with water; 4) eyes: saline or water irrigation

- Establish HIV status of source by history or rapid HIV test (with consent)
- Counseling HCW: 1) Risk (as summarized above); 2) risk for other bloodborne pathogens-HBV and HCV; 3) abstain or safe sex until serologic testing completed and negative
- HIV testing: 4th generation test that combines HIV p24 antigen-HIV antibody (preferred). Test at baseline, 6 weeks, and 4 months.
- Medical treatment within 72 hours.(effectiveness presumably declines with each hour of delay (CDC MMWR 2005; 54 (RR2:1-20):

Need for Expert Consultations (Call: PEPline 888-448-4911)

- 1) Delayed exposure report (>72 hrs); 2) unkown source; 3) known or suspected pregnancy; 4) breast feeding exposed person; 5) suspected HIV resistance in exposed person; 6) toxicity to PEP regimen; 7) serious medical condition in infected source.

TABLE 56: **Non-Occupational Post·Exposure Prophylaxis (PEP)**

Criteria for exposure: Exposure to source with known HIV infection or high risk (MSM, IVDU, sex worker)

Exposed site: Mucous membrane (vagina, rectum, mouth, eye), non intact skin or percutaneous

Exposure to: Blood or bloody fluid, vaginal or rectal secretions, or breast milk

Risk-Single exposure from infected source (CDC MMWR 2005 RR02; 54; Varghese B. Sex Transm Dis 2002; 29:37)

1) 3-5/1000: Needle-sharing IVDU, percutaneous needle stick
2) 0.1-1/1000: Receptive or insertive vaginal intercourse, receptive anal intercourse
3) 0.05-0.1/1000: Receptive oral intercourse

Timing: Medical treatment within 72 hours

Regimen: as for occupational exposure (see Table 57, page 105)

TABLE 56 CONTINUED

Laboratory testing of source: STDs, HBV, HCV and HIV; if HIV positive: resistance test, VL, CD4 count

Laboratory testing of the exposed person: HIV serology, CBC, LFTs, Scr, BUN, HBV, HCV, STDs

Post-exposure monitoring:

- HIV test of exposed person:

4th generation test with HIV p24 Ag and HIV Ab (preferred for early detection): baseline, 6 weeks, and 4 months or with any symptoms suggesting acute HIV infection. P24 Ag should be deteced at about 8-10 days. HIV RNA will be detected earlier.

3rd generation test: baseline, 6 weeks, 3 months, and 6 months

Report any seroconversion to CDC at 1-800-893-0485

TABLE 57: PEP Recommended Regimens

	Regimen (4 week duration)
Preferred	RAL 400 mg bid OR DTG* 50 mg qd plus TDF/FTC 300/200 mg qd
Alternative	DRV/r 800/100 mg qd plus TDF/FTC 300/200 mg qd
Other possible options	EVG/COBI/TDF/FTC (if CrCL >70 ml/min) ATV/r plus TDF/FTC RPV plus TDF/FTC LPV/r plus TDF/FTC

* Dolutegravir-based regimen added by authors reflecting current data for this agent which became FDA approved after publication of these PEP guidelines.

TABLE 58: PEP Toxicity Monitoring

Test	Baseline	Sx*	Wk 4-6	Wk 12	Wk 24
HIV EIA or rapid test	+	+	+	+	+
CBC, LFTs, and creatinine	+	+*	-	-	-
HIV viral load	-	+*	-	-	-
HBsAb	+	-	-	-	-
HBsAg	+	-	-	-	-
HCV Ab†	+	-	-	+	+

* Symptoms of drug toxicity or seroconversion syndrome

† Data on source and HBsAb status of host determines risk

Resources for PEP

- **PEPline:**
  http://nccc.ucsf.edu/
  Telephone: 1-888-448-4911--

- **Hepatitis Hotline:**
  Telephone: 1-888-443-7232

- **Report Occupational Exposure with Transmission: CDC guidance**
  Telephone: 1-800-893-0485 or 404-639-2050

- **HIV Pregnancy registry:**
  http://www.apregistry.com/
  Telephone: 1-800-258-4263
  Email: registry@nc.crl.com

- **HIV/AIDS Treatment Information Service:**
  http://aidsinfo.nih.gov/

BLE 59: **Pre-Exposure Prophylaxis (PrEP) (2014 CDC Recommendtions)**

(http://www.cdc.gov/hiv/pdf/prepguidelines2014.pdf) Clinical Provider's supplement (http://www.cdc.gov/hiv/pdf/prepprovidersupplement2014.pdf)

Indications

Indications: MSM

1) Adult male; 2) no acute or chronic HIV infection; 3) male sex partner in past 6 months;
4) not in a monogamous relationship with recently tested HIV negative man

PLUS

1) Anal sex without condoms in past 6 months; 2) any sexually transmitted infection diagnosed or reported in past 6 months; OR 3) in ongoing sexual relationship with HIV positive male partner.

Indications: Heterosexual men and women

1) Adult; 2) no acute or chronic HIV infection; 3) any heterosexual sex in past 6 months;
4) not in monogamous relationship with recently tested HIV negative partner

AND at least one of the following:

1) Infrequent use of condoms with one or more partners with unknown HIV status who are at "substantial HIV risk" (IDU or bisexual male); 2) in ongoing sexual relationship with HIV positive partner.

Indications: Injection drug users (IDUs)

1) Adult; 2) no acute or chronic HIV infection; 3) injection of drugs not physican prescribed in past 6 months

PLUS one of the following:

1) Sharing injection or drug preparation equipment in past 6 months; 2) been in a methadone, buprenorphine or suboxone treatment program in past 6 months; OR 3) risk of sexual transmission of HIV (see above)

Recommended oral PrEP medications

Regimen: TDF/FTC 300/200 mg po once daily. Note: TAF/FTC not recommended.
Time to Protection: Estimated at 7 days for rectal sex and 20 days for vaginal sex (based on tissue concentrations)
Monitoring Every 3 months: 1) HIV test; 2) refills for no more than 3 months; 3) pregnancy test for conception vulnerable q 3 months; 4) support for adherence and risk prevention;
5) assess side effects, adherence, risk behavior
Monitoring Every 6 months: 1) declining CrCL but > 60ml/min -- consult nephrologist; 2) test for sexually transmitted disease if sexually active -- syphilis, gonorrhea, *Chlamydia trachomatis*.
Drug interactions: TDF: possible increases of either TDF or interacting drug: acyclovir, valacyclovir, cidofovir, ganciclovir, valganciclovir; drugs that reduce renal function, including aminoglycoside, high-dose or multiple NSAIDs.
FTC: no data with drugs listed above, but interaction unlikely

Risk reduction counseling

Establish trust and communication
Support risk reduction efforts
Monitor behavioral adherence in non-judgmental manner

"As needed Coitally Dependent PrEP"
The IPERGAY trial tested the efficacy of TDF/FTC given prophylactically prior and after the time of anticipated sex in a high risk population of seronegatvie MSM who had frequent sex. The TDF/FTC vs. placebo controlled trial showed that prophylaxis using the regimen described below was 86% effective ($p<0.01$) in preventing HIV transmission

The regimen: 2 TDF/FTC (Truvada) pills at 2-24 hrs before sex (or one pill if the last dose was 1-6 days previously) and 2 doses 24 and 48 hrs after the pre-sex dose.

Note: TAF/FTC not recommended.

"Transition PrEP" or "Bridge PrEP":
This method employs PrEP in the standard TDF/FTC regimen (1 pill/day) for discordant couples in which the uninfected partner uses PrEP regimen during the period required by the infected partner to achieve viral suppression with ART.

The CDC issued a statement 2/24/15 urging people at "substantial risk" for HIV infection to take steps to reduce this risk by encouraging PrEP by MSM, heterosexual men and women and IDUs (CDC statement 2/24/15 http://cdc.gov/nchhstp/newsroom/2015/IPERGAY-2015-Media-Statement.html

Risk reduction counseling
Establish trust and communication
Support risk reduction efforts
Monitor behavioral adherence in non-judgmental manner

TABLE 60: **Dosing of antimicrobial agents for Patients with Chronic Kidney Disease (CKD) or End-Stage Renal Disease (ESRD).**

Adapted from Clinical Practice Guideline for the Management of Chronic Kidney Disease in Patients Infected with HIV: 2014 HIVMA/IDSA CID 2014.

Drug, dosing category	Dosage
Abacavir	
No dose adjustment with CKD or ESRD	600 mg po q24h or 300 mg po q12h
Acyclovir	
Cr CL > 50 mL/min	Usual dosage (high dose for zoster): 200–800 mg po 3-5 times per day; 5–10 mg per kg of ideal body weight IV q8h
Cr CL 25-50 mL/min	200-800 mg po 3-5 times per day; 5-10 mg/kg IV q12h
Cr CL 10-24 mL/min	200-800 mg po q8h; 5-10 mg/kg IV q24h
Cr CL < 10 mL/min	200-800 mg q12h; 2.5–5 mg per kg of ideal body weight IV q24h
Cr CL < 10 mL/min receiving hemodialysis	2.5–5 mg per kg of ideal body weight IV q24h. On days of HD, dose post-HD.
Amikacin	
Cr CL > 60 mL/min	Mycobacterial Infections: 15 mg/kg/d IV or 25 mg/kg TIW
Cr CL < 60 mL/min	Adjust dose based on serum concentrations. Target peak 35–45 mcg/mL and trough <4 mcg/mL.
Amphotericin B deoxycholate	
Cr CL > 50 mL/min	Usual dosage: 0.7-1.0 mg/kg iv q24h
Dosage for patients with CKD or ESRD	No dose adjustment (but consider lipid amphotericin formulations, azoles, or echinocandins)
Amphotericin B liposomal	
Cr CL > 50 mL/min	Usual dosage: 4.0–6.0 mg per kg of actual body weight iv q24h
Dosage for patients with CKD or ESRD	No dose adjustment

TABLE 60: **Dosing of antimicrobial agents for Patients with Chronic Kidney Disease (CKD) or End-Stage Renal Disease (ESRD).**

Drug, dosing category	Dosage
Atazanavir	
No dose adjustment with CKD or ESRD	ATV/r 300/100 mg once-daily or ATV 400 mg once-daily
Receiving hemodialysis	Avoid unboosted ATV Avoid boosted ATV in treatment-experienced patients with PI resistant mutations.
Azithromycin	
No dose adjustment with CKD or ESRD	MAC prophylaxis: 1200 mg once weekly MAC treatment: 500-600 mg once-daily (in combination with ethambutol +/- third drug)
Ceftriaxone	
No dose adjustment with CKD or ESRD	1-2 gm IM or IV once-daily GC: 250 mg IM x 1 Meningitis: 2 gm IV q12h
Cidofovir	
Cr CL > 55 mL/min and a urine protein < 100 mg/dL	Usual dosage: 5 mg per/kg IV q week x 2 weeks, then every other week (with probenecid and hydration)
Increase in serum creatinine level to 0.3–0.4 above baseline	3 mg per kg of body weight iv every other week (with probenecid and hydration)
Increase in serum creatinine level to ≥0.5 above baseline or development of grade 3+ proteinuria	Discontinue
Baseline serum creatinine level >1.5, creatinine clearance ≤55 mL/min, or grade ≥2+ proteinuria	Not recommended
Ciprofloxacin	
Cr CL > 50 mL/min	Usual dosage: 500-750 mg po q12h OR 400 IV q8h-12h
Cr CL 30–50 mL/min	500-750 mg q12h OR 400 IV q12h
Cr CL < 30 mL/min	250–500 mg q18-24h OR 400 IV q24h
Receiving hemodialysis	250–500 mg q24h OR 200-400 IV q24h (days of HD dose post-HD)

TABLE 60: **Dosing of antimicrobial agents for Patients with Chronic Kidney Disease (CKD) or End-Stage Renal Disease (ESRD).**

Drug, dosing category	Dosage	
Clarithromycin		
Cr CL > 30 mL/min	Usual dosage: 500 mg po q12h With ATV co-administration, reduce clarithromycin dose by 50%. With other PI co-administration, dose reduction by 50% with CrCL 30-60 mL/min.	
Cr CL < 30 mL/min	Reduce dose by one-half if creatinine clearance <30 mL/min. With PI co-administration, 75% reduction with CrCL <30 mL/min	
Dapsone		
No dose adjustment with CKD or ESRD	PCP prophylaxis: 100 mg once-daily PCP treatment (mild to moderate disease): 100 mg once-daily (in combination with trimethoprim)	
Daclatasvir		
No dose adjustment with CKD or ESRD	60 mg po once-daily (in combination with sofosbuvir)	
Darunavir		
No dose adjustment with CKD or ESRD	DRV/r 800/100 mg once-daily or DRV/r 600/100 mg twice-daily	
Didanosine EC		
Cr CL ≥ 60 mL/min	Body weight >60 kg	400 mg q24h
Cr CL 30–59 mL/min		200 mg q24h
Cr CL 10–29 mL/min		125 mg q24h
Cr CL < 10 mL/min		125 mg q24h
Receiving HD or PD		125 mg q24h
Cr CL ≥ 60 mL/min	Body weight <60 kg	250 mg q24h
Cr CL 30–59 mL/min		125 mg q24h
Cr CL 10–29 mL/min		125 mg q24h
Cr CL < 10 mL/min		75 mg (pediatric powder for suspension) q24h
Receiving HD or PD		75 mg (pediatric powder for suspension) q24h

TABLE 60: **Dosing of antimicrobial agents for Patients with Chronic Kidney Disease (CKD) or End-Stage Renal Disease (ESRD).**

Drug, dosing category	Dosage
Dolutegravir	
Cr CL > 30 ml/min	50 mg once-daily (ARV- or INSTI-naïve patients) 50 mg twice-daily (INSTI-experienced with certain INSTI mutations)
Cr CL < 30 ml/min	Use usual dose (above). DTG concentrations decreased by 40%. Clinical significance unknown, but INSTI-experienced patients with INSTI mutations may be at increased risk for virologic breakthrough.
Doxycycline	
No dose adjustment with CKD or ESRD	100 mg po twice-daily
Efavirenz	
No dose adjustment with CKD or ESRD	600 mg po qhs
Elvitegravir	
No dose adjustment with CKD when combined with boosted PI	EVG 85 mg once-daily + ATV/r 300/100 mg once-daily EVG 150 mg once-daily + DRV/r 600/100 mg twice-daily
Cr CL ≥ 70 mL/min	EVG/COBI/TDF/FTC 150/150/300/200 mg (Stribild) 1 tablet po q24h. D/C if Cr CL < 50 ml/min.
Cr CL ≥ 30 mL/min	EVG/COBI/TAF/FTC 150/150/10/200 mg tablet once daily; discontinue if CrCL <30mL/min
Emtricitabine	
Cr CL ≥ 50 mL/min	200 mg po q24h
Cr CL 30–49 mL/min	200 mg po q48h
Cr CL 15–29 mL/min	200 mg po q 3 days
Cr CL < 15 mL/min	200 mg po q 4 days
Receiving hemodialysis	200 mg po q 4 days
Receiving peritoneal dialysis	No data. Dose reduction needed
Enfuvirtide	
No dose adjustment with CKD or ESRD	90 mg subcutaneous twice-daily

TABLE 60: **Dosing of antimicrobial agents for Patients with Chronic Kidney Disease (CKD) or End-Stage Renal Disease (ESRD).**

Drug, dosing category	Dosage
Entecavir	
Cr CL ≥ 50 mL/min	0.5 mg q24h (HBV treatment-naïve); 1 mg q24h (3TC-refractory HBV or with decompensated liver disease)
Cr CL 30-49 mL/min	0.25 mg q24h (HBV treatment-naïve); 0.5 mg q24h (3TC-refractory HBV or with decompensated liver disease)
Cr CL 10-29 mL/min	0.15 mg q24h (HBV treatment-naïve); 0.3 mg q24h (3TC-refractory HBV or with decompensated liver disease)
Cr CL < 10 mL/min; HD or PD	0.05 mg q24h or 0.5 mg q7d (HBV treatment-naïve); 0.1 mg q24h or 1 mg q7d (3TC-refractory HBV or with decompensated liver disease)
Ethambutol	
Cr CL > 50 mL/min	Usual dosage: 15–25 mg per kg of body weight po q24h
Cr CL 10–50 mL/min	15–25 mg per kg of body weight po q24–36h
Cr CL < 10 mL/min	15–25 mg per kg of body weight po q48h
Etravirine	
No dose adjustment with CKD or ESRD	200 mg po twice-daily
Famciclovir	
Cr CL > 40 mL/min	Usual dosage: 500 mg po q12h (HSV); 500 q8h (VZV)
Cr CL 20–39 mL/min	500 mg q24h
Cr CL < 20 mL/min	250 mg q24h
Receiving hemodialysis	250 mg after each dialysis
Fluconazole	
Cr CL > 50 mL/min	Usual dosage: 200-1200 mg po q24h
Cr CL = or < 50 mL/min	1/2 dose
Receiving hemodialysis	Full dose after dialysis

TABLE 60: **Dosing of antimicrobial agents for Patients with Chronic Kidney Disease (CKD) or End-Stage Renal Disease (ESRD).**

Drug, dosing category		Dosage
Flucytosine Monitor concentrations: target 30-80 mcg/mL (2hr post dose)		
Cr CL > 40 mL/min		Usual dosage: 25mg/kg q6h
Cr CL 20-40 mL/min		25 mg/kg q12h
Cr CL 10-20 mL/min		25 mg/kg q24h
Cr CL < 10 mL/min		25 mg/kg q48h
Fosamprenavir		
No dose adjustment with CKD or ESRD		FPV/r 1400/100 mg once-daily or FPV/r 700/100 mg twice-daily
Foscarnet IV		
CrCl (mL/min/kg)	CMV Induction Treatment	CMV Maintenance Treatment
>1.4	90mg/kg q12h	90 mg/kg q24h
1.0-1.4	70 mg/kg q12h	70 mg/kg q24h
0.8-1.0	50 mg/kg q12h	50 mg/kg q24h
0.6-0.8	80 mg/kg q24h	80 mg/kg q48h
0.5-0.6	60 mg/kg q24h	60 mg/kg q48h
0.4-0.5	50 mg/kg q24h	50 mg/kg q48h
<0.4	Not recommended	Not recommended
Ganciclovir IV		
Usual dosage		5mg/kg q12h (induction [I]); 5mg/kg q24h(maintenance [M])
50-69 mL/min		2.5 mg/kg q12h (I); 2.5 mg/kg q24h (M)
25-49 mL/min		2.5 mg/kg q24h (I); 1.25 mg/kg q24h (M)
10-24 mL/min		1.25 mg/kg q24h (I); 0.625 mg/kg q24h (M)
< 10 mL/min; HD		1.25 mg/kg TIW (I) post-HD; 0.625 mg/kg TIW (M) post-HD
Indinavir		
No dose adjustment with CKD or ESRD		IDV/r 800/100 mg po twice-daily

TABLE 60: **Dosing of antimicrobial agents for Patients with Chronic Kidney Disease (CKD) or End-Stage Renal Disease (ESRD).**

Drug, dosing category	Dosage	
Isoniazid		
Cr CL > 10 mL/min	Usual dosage: 300 mg po q24h	
Cr CL < 10 mL/min	300 mg q24h (on days of HD, dose post-HD); consider dose adjustment in slow acetylators.	
Itraconazole		
No dose adjustment with CKD or ESRD	Candida esophagitis: 200 mg liquid once-daily Coccidioidomycosis: 200 mg twice-daily Target peak (2hr post-dose): > 1 mcg/mL	
Lamivudine		
Cr CL > 50 mL/min	300 mg po q 24h or 150 mg po q12h	
Cr CL 30–49 mL/min	150 mg po q 24h	
Cr CL 15–29 mL/min	150 mg po first dose, then 100 mg po q 24h	
Cr CL 5–14 mL/min	150 mg po first dose, then 50 mg* po q24h.	*To avoid using the liquid formulation and because of the favorable safety profile, the authors use lowest available tablet dose of 100 mg (lamivudine HB) or 150 mg (lamivudine) daily
Cr CL < 5mL/min, hemodialysis, or peritoneal dialysis	50 mg po first dose, then 25 mg* po q24h.	
Levofloxacin		
Cr CL > 50 mL/min	Usual dosage: 500–750 mg IV or po q24h	
Cr CL 20-49 mL/min	500mg loading dose, then 250 mg q24h	
Cr CL 10-19 mL/min	500mg loading dose, then 250 mg q48h	
Receiving hemodialysis or PD	750-500 mg loading dose, then 250-500 mg q48h (dose post-HD on days of dialysis)	
Lopinavir/ritonavir		
No dose adjustment with CKD or ESRD	400 mg/100 mg po twice-daily. OR 800 mg/200 mg po once-daily	
Receiving hemodialysis	LPV trough lower in HD, use with caution in patients with PI resistant mutations.	

TABLE 60: **Dosing of antimicrobial agents for Patients with Chronic Kidney Disease (CKD) or End-Stage Renal Disease (ESRD).**

Drug, dosing category	Dosage
Maraviroc	
Cr CL > 30 mL/min	300 mg po twice-daily
Cr CL < 30 mL/min	300 mg po twice-daily Reduce dose to 150 mg po twice-daily if orthostatic hypotension occurs. Avoid MVC with CYP3A4 inhibitor (e.g. macrolides, protease inhibitors).
Metronidazole	
No dose adjustment with CKD or ESRD	250-500 mg q8h *C. difficile* colitis: 500 mg po q8h x 10-14 days BV or Trichomonas: 500 mg po q12h x 7 days
Moxifloxacin	
No dose adjustment with CKD or ESRD	400 mg po or IV once-daily
Nelfinavir	
No dose adjustment with CKD or ESRD	1250 mg po twice-daily or 750 mg q8h
Nevirapine	
No dose adjustment with CKD or ESRD	Usual dose: 200 mg po twice-daily (after 2 weeks of 200 mg po once-daily)
Nitazoxanide	
No dose adjustment with CKD or ESRD	Cryptosporidiosis: 0.5-1.0 gm po twice-daily (in combination with ART)
Paritaprevir (150 mg)/Ritonavir (100 mg)/Ombitasvir (25 mg) and Dasabuvir (250 mg)	
No dose adjustment with CKD or ESRD	Paritaprevir (150 mg)/Ritonavir (100 mg)/Ombitasvir (25 mg) once-daily + Dasabuvir (250 mg) twice-daily.
Paromomycin	
No dose adjustment with CKD or ESRD	Cryptosporidiosis: 500 mg po q6h (in combination with ART)

TABLE 60: **Dosing of antimicrobial agents for Patients with Chronic Kidney Disease (CKD) or End-Stage Renal Disease (ESRD).**

Drug, dosing category	Dosage
Penicillin G	
Cr CL > 50 mL/min	Streptococcal endocarditis, neurosyphilis or ocular syphilis: 3–4 MU IV q4h OR 18–24 MU continuous IV infusion daily
Cr CL 10-50 mL/min	2–3 MU IV q4h OR 12–18 MU continuous IV infusion daily.
Cr CL < 10 mL/min	2 MU IV q4–6h OR 8–12 MU continuous IV infusion daily.
Receiving HD or PD	2 MU IV q6h OR 8 MU continuous IV infusion daily.
Pentamidine	
Cr CL > 50 mL/min	Usual dosage: 4.0 mg per kg of body weight IV q24h
Cr CL 10–50 mL/min	3.0 mg per kg of body weight IV q24h (use with caution)
Cr CL < 10 mL/min	4.0 mg per kg of body weight iv q-48h
Posaconazole	
Cr CL > 50 mL/min	Esophageal candidiasis (refractory to fluconazole and itraconazole): 400 mg po q12h Invasive fungal infections: 300 mg IV q12h x 2 (load), then 300 mg IV once-daily, then transition to oral posaconazole once clinically stable (400 mg po twice-daily; up to 1200 mg/day). Target trough for invasive infections > 1.25 mcg/mL
Cr CL < 50 mL/min	Usual oral posaconazole dose Large pharmacokinetlc variability with Cr CL < 20 mL/min. Use with close monitoring. Avoid IV posaconazole because of potential toxicity due to accumulation of sulfobutylether-cyclodexrin (SBECD vehicle of IV product). Based on observational study with IV voriconazole, this appears to be not a genuine concern.

TABLE 60: **Dosing of antimicrobial agents for Patients with Chronic Kidney Disease (CKD) or End-Stage Renal Disease (ESRD).**

Drug, dosing category	Dosage
Pyrazinamide	
Cr CL > 10 mL/min	Usual dosage: 20–25 mg/kg (max 2 gm) po q24h
Cr CL < 10 mL/min	50% of usual dose
Receiving hemodialysis	Usual dose post-HD
Pyrimethamine	
No dose adjustment with CKD or ESRD	Toxoplasmosis treatment: 200 mg x 1, then 50 mg (<60 kg) or 75 mg (> 60 kg) po once-daily (in combination sulfadiazine or clindamycin)
Raltegravir	
No dose adjustment with CKD or ESRD	400 mg po twice-daily
Ribavirin	
Cr CL > 50 mL/min	Usual dosage: 800-1200 mg/day po in two divided doses.
Cr CL 30-50 mL/min	Alternate 200 mg and 400 mg every other day.
Cr CL < 30 mL/min	200 mg po qd
Cr CL < 10 mL/min on HD	200mg/d (limited data w/ high dropout rates)
Rifabutin	
Cr CL > 30 mL/min	Usual dosage: 300 mg po q24h (dose adjustment needed with PI/r or PI/c co-administration)
Cr CL < 30 mL/min	Consider 50% dose reduction
Rifampin	
Cr CL > 50 mL/min	Usual dosage: 600 mg po q24h
Cr CL 10–50 mL/min	100% of full dose
Cr CL < 10 mL/min	50%–100% of full dose
Receiving hemodialysis	50%–100% of full dose; no supplement
Receiving peritoneal dialysis	50%–100% of full dose; extra 50%–100% of full dose after receipt of peritoneal dialysis. TDM recommended

TABLE 60: **Dosing of antimicrobial agents for Patients with Chronic Kidney Disease (CKD) or End-Stage Renal Disease (ESRD).**

Drug, dosing category	Dosage	
Rilpivirine		
No dose adjustment with CKD or ESRD	25 mg po once-daily	
Cr CL ≥ 30 mL/min	RPV/TAF/FTC 25/25/200 mg tablet once daily with food; discontinue if CrCL <30mL/min	
Saquinavir		
No dose adjustment with CKD or ESRD	SQV/r 1000/100 mg po twice-daily	
Simeprevir		
No dose adjustment with CKD or ESRD	150 mg po once-daily (in combination with sofosbuvir)	
Sofosbuvir		
Cr CL > 30 mL/min	400 mg po once-daily (in combination with another HCV agent)	
Cr CL < 30 mL/min	Dose not established. Up to 20-fold higher sofosbuvir metabolite observed in ESRD. Clinical significance unknown.	
Sofosbuvir-Ledipasvir		
Cr CL > 30 mL/min	Sofosbuvir/Ledipasvir 400/90 mg po once-daily	
Cr CL < 30 mL/min	Dose not established. Ledipasvir concentrations unlikely to be affected. Up to 20-fold increase in sofosbuvir metabolite in ESRD. Clinical significance unknown.	
Stavudine		
Cr CL > 50 mL/min	30 mg po q12h	The FDA recommends a higher dose in patients who are > 60 kg, but this is associated with higher rates of toxicities (peripheral neuropathy, mitochondria toxicity, lactic acidosis).
Cr CL 26–50 mL/min	15 mg po q12h	
Cr CL ≤25 mL/min	15 mg po q24h	
Receiving hemodialysis	15 mg po q24h	
Receiving peritoneal dialysis	No data. Dose reduction recommended.	

TABLE 60: **Dosing of antimicrobial agents for Patients with Chronic Kidney Disease (CKD) or End-Stage Renal Disease (ESRD).**

Drug, dosing category	Dosage
Streptomycin	
Cr CL > 60 mL/min	MDRTB: 15 mg/kg IM q24h OR 25 mg/kg IM TIW
Cr CL < 60 mL/min	Use with caution. Adjust dose based on levels. Target trough < 10 mcg/mL
Sulfadiazine	
Cr CL > 50 mL/min	Usual dosage: 1-1.5 gm po q6h (1.5g for >60kg)
Tenofovir alafenamide + emtricitabine	
Cr CL ≥ 30 mL/min	TAF/FTC 25/200 mg tab once daily
Cr CL < 30 mL/min	Avoid
Tenofovir DF	
Cr CL ≥ 50 mL/min	300 mg po q24h
Cr CL 30–49 mL/min	300 mg po q48h
Cr CL 10–29 mL/min	300 mg po q72-96h
Receiving hemodialysis	300 mg po every 7 days (an additional dose may be needed if >12h HD per week)
Receiving peritoneal dialysis	No data. Dose reduction recommended.
Tenofovir/Emtricitabine	
Cr CL ≥ 50 mL/min	300 /200 mg po q24h
Cr CL 30–49 mL/min	300/200 mg po q48h
Cr CL < 30 mL/min	Coformulation not recommended. See TDF and FTC dosing recs.
Trimethoprim	
Cr CL > 30 mL/min	Usual dosage (mild to moderate PCP treatment): 5 mg/kg po q6–8h (in combination with dapsone)
Cr CL 10–30 mL/min	5 mg per kg po q12h (in combination with dapsone)
Cr CL < 10 mL/min	5 mg per kg po q24h (in combination with dapsone)

TABLE 60: **Dosing of antimicrobial agents for Patients with Chronic Kidney Disease (CKD) or End-Stage Renal Disease (ESRD).**

Drug, dosing category	Dosage
Trimethoprim sulfamethoxazole	PCP prophylaxis
Cr CL > 30 mL/min	Usual dosage (PCP prophylaxis): 1 double strength dose po q24h; 1 double strength dose po 3 times per week; 1 single strength dose po q24h
Cr CL 15–30 mL/min	1/2 dose
Cr CL < 15 mL/min	1/2 dose or use alternative agent
Trimethoprim sulfamethoxazole	PCP treatment
Cr CL > 30 mL/min	Usual dosage (PCP treatment): 5 mg/kg (as TMP component) IV or po q6–8h (+ steroid with Pao2 < 70 mm Hg or A-a gradient > 35 mm Hg
Cr CL 10–30 mL/min	5 mg per kg IV or po (as TMP component) q12h
Cr CL < 10 mL/min	5 mg per kg IV or po (as TMP component) q24h
Valacyclovir	
Cr CL > 50 mL/min	Usual dosage: 500 mg–1g po q8h
Cr CL 30-49 mL/min	500 mg–1g po q12h
Cr CL 10-20 mL/min	500-1 g mg po q24h
Cr CL < 10 mL/min	500 mg po q24h

TABLE 60: **Dosing of antimicrobial agents for Patients with Chronic Kidney Disease (CKD) or End-Stage Renal Disease (ESRD).**

Drug, dosing category	Dosage
Valganciclovir	
Cr CL > 50 mL/min	Usual dosage: 900 mg po q12h (induction); 900 mg po q24h (maintenance)
Cr CL 40–59 mL/min	450 mg q12h (induction); 450 mg q24h (maintenance).
Cr CL 25–39 mL/min	450 mg q.d.(induction); 450 mg q48h (maintenance)
Cr CL 10–24 mL/min	450 mg q48h (induction); 450 mg twice per week (maintenance).
Cr CL < 10 mL/min	Not recommended by US manufacturer. Use IV ganciclovir or consider 200 mg suspension TIW (induction)/ 100 mg suspension TIW (maintenance).
Receiving hemodialysis	Consider 200 mg oral powder formulation TIW (induction); 100 mg TIW (maintenance)
Voriconazole	
Cr CL > 50 ml/min	Aspergillosis: 6 mg/kg IV q12h x 2 (load), then 4 mg/kg q12h. Target trough > 2.05 mcg/mL Candidemia: 6 mg/kg IV q12h x 2 (load), then 3 mg/kg IV q12h Oral once clinically stable: 200–300 mg po q12h
Cr CL < 50 mL/min	Usual oral dose Avoid IV voriconazole because of potential toxicity due to accumulation of sulfobutylether-cyclodexrin (vehicle of IV product). Based on observational study this appears to be not a genuine concern.
Zidovudine	
Cr CL > 15 mL/min	Usual dose: 300 mg po q12h
Cr CL < 15 mL/min, HD, or PD	100 mg po q6-8h or 300 mg po q24h

NOTES

CPSIA information can be obtained
at www.ICGtesting.com
Printed in the USA
BVOW10s2150050616
450704BV00005B/15/P

9 780996 733304